Studies on the mechanism of binding of ^{99}Tc-MDP to human serum albumin

Prof. Dr. Sami A. Al-Mudhaffer

Dr. Abdul Husain Al-Jeboori

Contents in brief

Contents

Chapter 1
Introduction

1.1 GENERAL KNOWLEDEGE

1.1.1 isotopes in clinical chemistry:

The isotopic properties will make the labeled compound more easily identifiable. For example, the radioiodine – labeled thyroxine molecules can be identified and quantified easily by virtue of their radioactivity (1).

The use of isotopes, both stable and radioactive, has proved great body of information in the medical scince. Stable isotopes are non radioactive and are suitable for use as tracers in humans. Especially infants children and pregnant women, stable isotopes have also been used in the quantative analysis of various substances in recent years.

Radioactivity measurements depends on the ability of radionuclides to produce ionized or excited atoms within the detector (2). Two basic types of radiation detectors are in common use: gas ionization ans scintillation (2). Radioisotopes allow the detection of minute quantities and differenate physically between substances.

The use of radioactive isotopes in biochemistry and clinical chemistry has proved us with a wealth of information about biological processes, that offers such as adiverse range of applications, using enzyme assays, biochemical pathways of synthesis and degradation, analysis of biomolecules, measurement of antibodies, binding and transport studies (3).

The use of radionuclide in nuclear medicine began when Frederick proescher published the paper entitled the use of radium for therapy of various diseases (1). Early experimental and diagnostic applications were performed with naturally occurring radionuclides, then the radioisotope with physical short half loves have become increasingly popular for imaging applications (4).

The first commercially available radioisotope generator was the ^{132}Tc-^{132}I, (5) several other generators (such as Mo-^{99m}Tc, ^{68}GE-68Ga, ^{113}Sn-^{113}In, ^{87}Y-^{87m}Sr....etc) subsequently evolved (6-9). These generators must meet certain physical basic criteria to be useful. It should. It should be simple and convenient to operate, radiation must be adequately shielded------- yield adaughter product of high purity in terms of both radioactivity stable contaminants during every clution throughout the life of the generator, the product should be in a chemical form suitable for use with amininmum of additional chemical or physical manipulation, lastly the radioactive yield of the daughter product during each elution should be high (10, 11).

Labeled compounds either be used in biochemical research --- routine medical diagnosis were carried out in vivo for medical diagnosis such as those labeled with gamma emitting isotopes to permit detection external to the patient, (12) but those labeled with beta-emitting isotopes such as: ^{14}C, ^{3}H, ^{35}S and ^{32}P were principally used in biochemical research (13).

There are various methods which were used for preparing labeled compounds such as of the followings:

1- isotope exchange reactions, in which one or more atoms in the molecule, exchange with atoms of the same element and of different mass, these atoms may be radioactive or stable isotopes, according to the following:

$$AX^* + BX \rightarrow BX^* + AX$$

The compound BX under certain reaction conditions will exchange its X atom (s) with the compound AX^* where X^* atom (s) is an isotopic form of the element X. awide range of compounds labeled with different stable or radioactive isotopes are prepared by exchange methods, which have the advantage that they can normally be carred out on a small chemical scale. An example is the preparation of urea C, (14-15)

$$CO(NH_2)_2 + {}^{14}CO_2 \rightarrow {}^{14}CO(NH_2)_2 + CO$$

2- chemical synthesis in volves the construction of complex moleculry from simple isotopically labeled intermediates, yields are usually expre as a percentage radiochemical yield:

$$\% \text{Radiochemical yield} = \frac{\text{Total radioactivity in product}}{\text{Total radioactivity in substrate}} \times 100$$

For example, the preparation of carboxyl-labelled fatty acids by reaction with the corresponding grignard reagent or acetic anhydride- ${}^{14}C$, steroids ${}^{14}C$ and amino acids-${}^{14}C$ (16-19).

3- biochemical methods: these include different procedures such as enzymatic synthesis which isvery similar to chemical synthesis in that such aconversion usually occurs without any change in the specificity of the labeling or the molar specific activity (16). Total biosynthetic methods are normally of value only when microorganisms are employed, but the production of uniformly labeled carbohydrates by photosynthesis in detached leaves is an exception to this (17, 18).

4- recoil labeling (19, 20): this method depend on the ability of recoil atom produced in a nuclear reaction to form a stable bond with an organic (or an inorganic) compound. For example, if an organic compound is mixed with a lithium carbonate or chloride and irradiated in anuclear reactor at fixed neutron flux, tritium compounds are produced by the recoiling "tritons" from the nuclear reaction $^6Li(n, \alpha)^3H$

One of the most radioisotopes used in clinical application in both cases as pure radioisotope or in labeled compounds is technetium-99m, which have a short half-life about six hours, with a predominate single photon gama emission having an energy of 140 kev (21). ^{99m}Tc-labelled compounds are diagnostic imaging agents used in the field of unclear medicine to visualize tissue anatomical structures and metabolic disorders. After interavenous administration ^{99m}Tc or it labeled compounds localized in specific target organ or tissue, can then be imaged using stable instrument (22).

1.2 TECHNETIUM CHEMISTRY

Technetium is not a naturally abundant element, some of its properties were produced by mendeleev in 1869, who called it ekamangabese and gave it the symbol (EM) (23). After world war II, Perrier and segre gave element 43 the name technetium as the first artificial element (24).

Tc chemistry is similar to its neighbouring elements managanese and rhenium a comprehensive review on tc-chemistry was published by deutch et al (25) , some of physical properties of tc are shown in table (1.1)

Table (1.1): some of tc physical properties

Property	Value
Melting point	2250±50c
Density	11.5g / cm3
Atomic weight	98.913
Ionization potential	7.28 ev
Entropy of crystallization	7.4±0.2 e.u.
Critical temperature or super conducting	7.7 kelven
Stable electronic state	4s 4p 4d 5s

To give rise to multiple oxidation states an forms coordination complexes with avariety of inorganic and organic ligands (26). The chemistry of Tc in its I-V oxidation states was sureveyd by davison and jones, many of the thermodynamically stable Tc-complexes have oxygen bound to it like TcO4, $TcO_2.2H_2O$, Tc-O-Ligand (27-29). Tc V and IV complexes are knwn to have the ligand coordinated to the Tc alone, i.e Tc, Tc_2Ln....etc, the polyncuclear formation of Tc species is usually minimized by keeping the Tc-concentration as low as possible, to prevent the formation of Tc complexes with more than one oxidation state, efforts are made to control the reducing agent and the reaction conditions, Fig (1.1) show some of Tc-complexes at different oxidation stte (30).

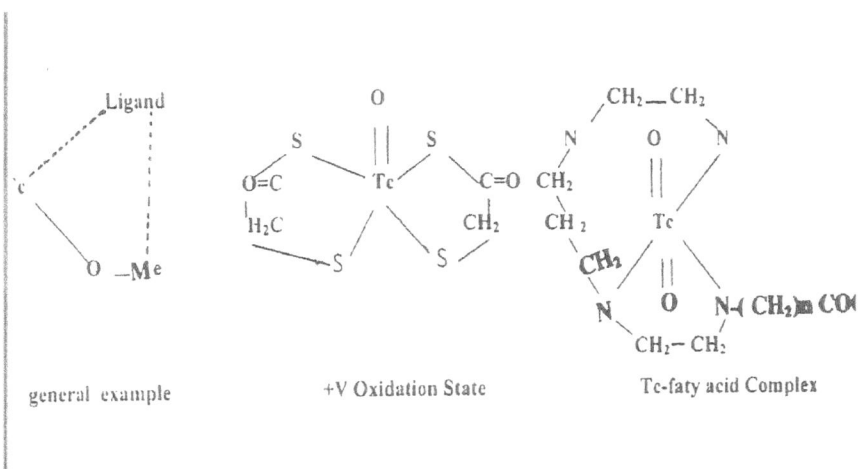

Fig(1.1)Some Tc-complexes at different oxidation state.

1.2.1 prouction of ^{99m}Tc

^{99m}Tc is usually produced from agenerator system as aresult of the decay of molybdenum ^{99m}Mo according to the following equation:

decay of molybdenum Mo according to the following equation:

$$^{99}Mo + n \Rightarrow ^{99}Mo \xrightarrow[67h]{\beta,\gamma} {}^{99m}Tc \xrightarrow[6h]{\gamma} {}^{99}Tc$$

Generators have been developed to take the advantage of this property and make ^{99m}Tc widely available in nuclear medicine laboratiries (31), the generator containing ^{99m}Mo as sodium molydate adsorbed onto an aluminium oxide column shown in fig (1.2), ^{99m}Tc is coninously formed by the decay of ^{99m}Mom elution of the column with isotonic saline yielded solution of pertechnetate which is chemically stable, sterile, pyrogen free and almost molybdenum and aluminium free (32, 33). Generators can either be ekuted by negative pressure, where there is astore of saline at the input to the column and an evacuated vial is placed over the outlet, or by positive pressure, where a quantity of saline is pushed through the column and the eluate collected in a sterile vial with needle attached.

^{99m}Mo is available from one of two sources, either from neutron bombardment of ^{99m}Mo in reactors (34), or from chemical separation of the fission products of uranium (235), (35) in this case all Mo in the form of ^{99m}Mo and the column itself can be made more efficient and eluted with a small volume of saline, thus a hiher specific activity eluted can be obtained which is usefull in various areas of clinical application (36).

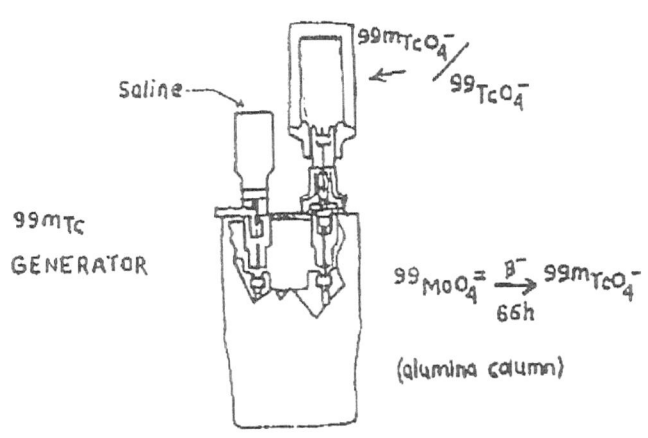

Fig(1.2) ^{99m}Tc-Generator.

1.2.2 principles of labeling with technetium :

The labeling of biologically important molecules with Tc means the introduction of a foreign element. Though the exact nature of the chemical bonding of Tc is still controversial, we can draw some important general conclusions from the viewpoint of periodic realationships (37).

Tc is amember of group VII B of the periodic table of the elements, thus belonging to the transition elements. Transition element are those hving partly filled (d) or (f) shells. Tc as an elements of the second series has partly filled 4d shells. The seven electrons in Tc (beyond the noble gas configuration) are easily stripped to yield Tc (VII) ((generator elute)) as the stable compound at the oxidation state +7 is the starting material for preparation of Tc-labelled compound (38, 39).

The principle of labeling has been shown to be complex formation (40-43). Tc in complexes is surrounded by anions or neutral molecules (ligand). Mono-denate ligands such as (F, CI, CN...) donate only one electron pair to the Tc atom, and its complexes with Tc are not stable in neutral aqueous solution. Multidanate ligands (chelate ligands) are suitable substances for labeling with Tc, as shown in table (1.2), complex formation occurs for compounds possessing functional group such as hydroxyl, carboxyl, amino, phosphate... etc. in appropriate molecular arrangement. Hence, using current labeling procedures, hydrophilic substabces that contain cheleate noietes are the predominat source of Tc-labelled compound. This implies preferable application of ionized biochemical and drugs (eg, hydroxycarboxylates, mercaptocarboxylates, phosphate compounds....etc) instead of pure ipophilic substance.

Tabe (1.2): some typical substances used for the preparation of ^{99m}Tc labelled compounds.

Substances	Functional group
Citrate	OH, COOH
Gkucinate	OH, COOH
Glucohephonate	OH, COOH
Sugars	OH
DTPA	COOH, IDA
Dimercaptosuccinate	SH, COOH
Mercaptoisobutyrate	SH, COOH
Penicillamine	SH, NH2, COOH
EHDP	OH , PO$_3$, H
MDP	PO$_3$, H
6-mercaptopurine	SH, arom, N

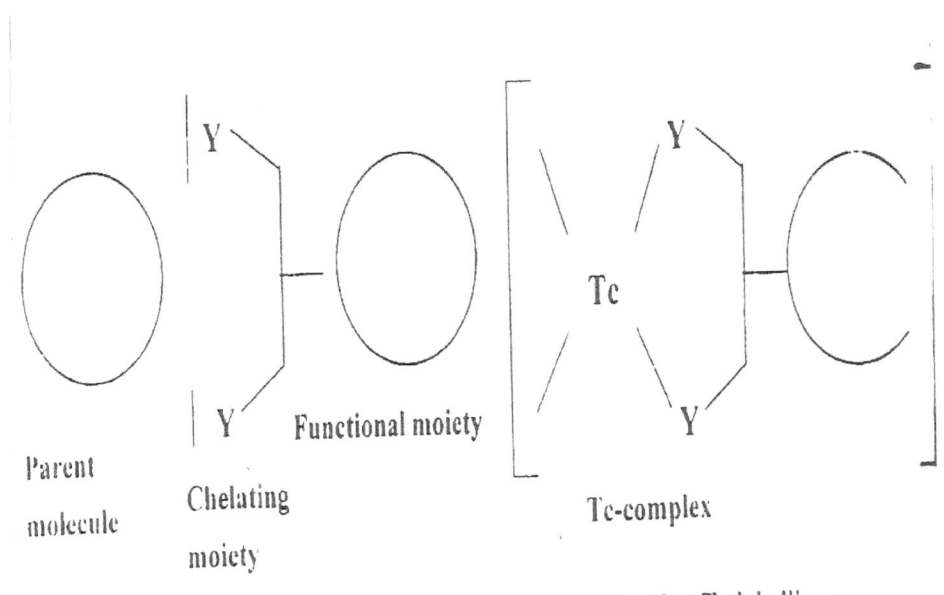

Parent
molecule

Chelating
moiety

Functional moiety

Tc-complex

Fig 1.3 The concept of bifunctional agents applied to Tc-labelling.

Initial applications of this approch have been reported to proteins and fatty acids(44,45).The complex of MDP with.Tc proved to be polymeric with technetium centres bridged by MDP and OH ligands(46) as shown in fig (1.4)

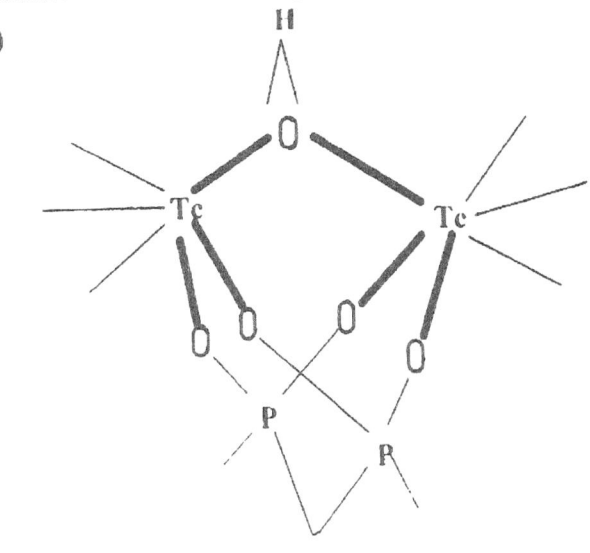

Fig (1.4): Polymeric Tc-OH-(MDP)$_n$

A general scheme in fig (1.5) Show the reactions which have to be considered in the preparation of ^{99m}Tc-labelled compound.

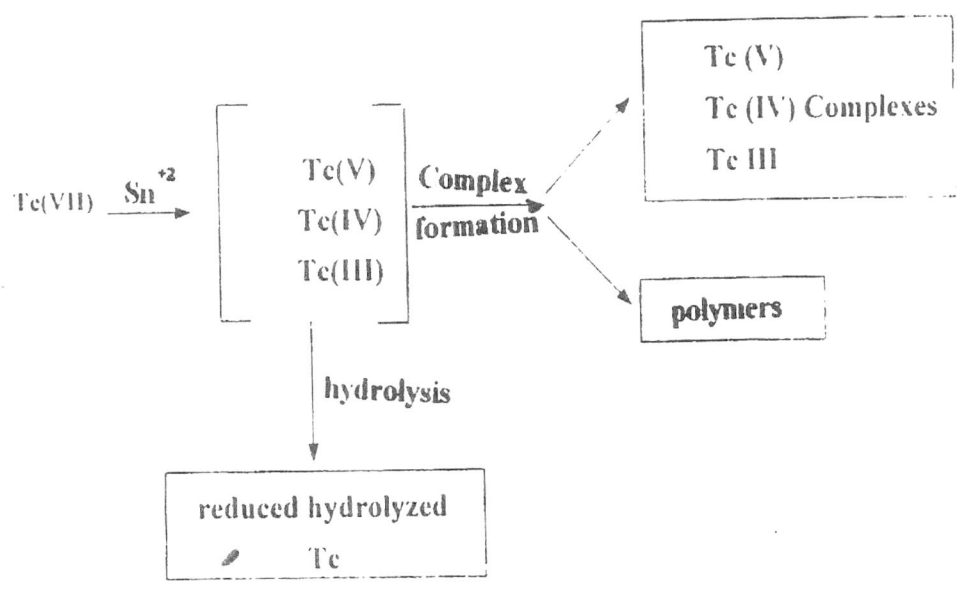

Fig(1.5):General scheme of ^{99m}Tc-labelled compound.

1.2.3 methods of detection:

^{99m}Tc can either be administrated to a patient as sodium pertechnetate, or it may be labelled with a range of compounds with avariety of useful biological distributions. The administeraed activity can be recoreded with appropriate radiation detectors such s scanners, gamma cameras, whole body imagers and renogram. All these detectors which can be utilized in a nuclear medicine basically acts as atransducer which transforms incoming eadiation into visible light (47) as in fig (1.6).

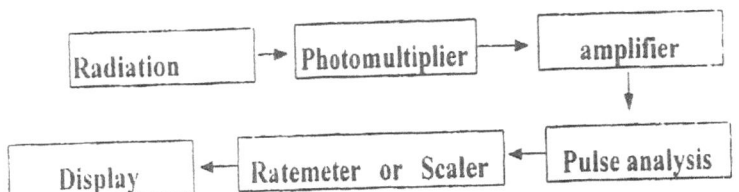

Fig(1.6) :Standard configuration of a radiation detector and display system.

The detection of radioactivity is carried out by one of the three following methods:

1- detecting areas of increased concentration of the radioisotope tracer within an area of relative homogeneous distribution of the labelled complex (hot spot imaging) as seen in brain tumours, bone metastases and myocardial infarction (48, 49). Fig (1.7) show one of these cases.

2- detecting areas of reduced concentration of the radioactive tracer within a uniform radioactive organ (cold sot imaging) as in liver tumours, renal nd thyroid cysts, (50 51) fig (1.8) show one of these cases.

3- monitoring the arrival and disappearance of the radioactivity over an area of interest ((time activity curves)) over the kidneys as in renography, fig (1.9) the brain as in cer bral perfusion studies or the heart as in left ventricular volume curves.

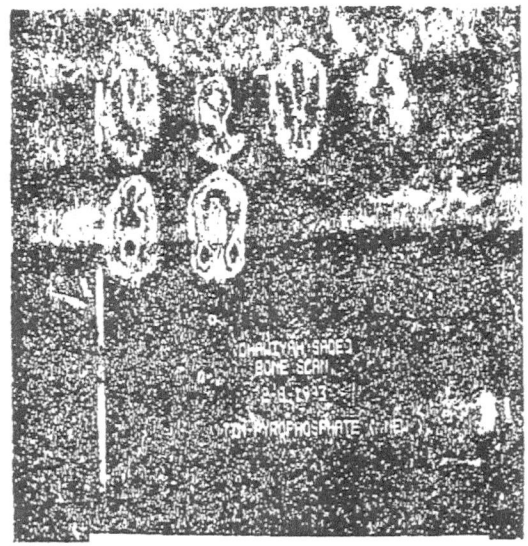

Fig(1.7) ^{99m}Tc-MDP-bone scanning .

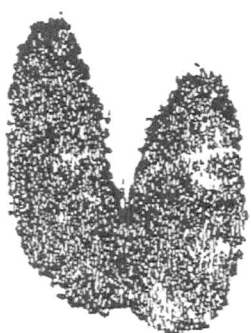

Fig(1.8).An image of a diffusely enlarged overacting thyroid typical of Graves disease .

1.3 ^{99m}TC-APPLICATION IN NUCLEAR MEDICINE

The following are some applications of ^{99m}Tc and its labelled compounds in unclear nedicine.

1.3.1 theroid imaging:

The trappng of ^{99m}Tc as sodium pertechnate by thyroid is useful for assessing both function and its anatomy of the gland (52), although thyroid gland requires iodide ion for the production of thyroxine and triodothyronine the iodide ions are transported across the memberans of the epithelial cells in the thyroid follicles by means of an active transport process, but the radius of iodide is comparable to that of pertechnetate and each of the ions has asingle negative charge then hey have asimilar charge densities, so that ^{99m}TcO4 is taken up readily by thyroid cells, evenm though iodine has several gamma-energies, so ^{99m}TcO4 is preferred (29).

1.3.2. brain imaging:

Its is limited to the detection of ruptures of tumours and vascular lesions that impair the function of the blood brain barrier which is normally impermeable to he highly water-soluble ^{99m}TcO$_4$ (53). The rate at which substances penetrate brain tissue through the blood-brain barier is inversely related to their size and directly related to their lipid solubility (54), therefore attempts have been made to design small Tc-complexes with hydrophobic ligands such as bis-aminoethanethiol, propylene amine oxime (55). Each of these agents readily croses the blood brain barier but subsequently clears the brain tissue in a matter of minutes due to the lack of affinity for any particular recptor sites to these agents (56, 57).

1.3.3. kidney imaging:

Nearly all ^{99m}Tc –labelled compound will be excreted by the kidneys and eliminated in the urine, becaue of the kidneys are the principle organ responsible for the exceretion of water-oluble substances from the body the functional unit of the kidney is called the nephron, it is composed of afiltering apparatus referred to as the glomerulus, which is encapsulated in a structure called the bowman's capsule, following the glomerulus is a multisegmented tubule system which reabsorbs nutrients and secrets unwanted substances (58). Dynamic imaging of the glomerular filleration process is normally carried out with tc-DTPA (T-diethyl enetriamine penta acetic) (59,60), the tc DTPA) readily passes through the glomerular filtration apparatus and because it is not reabsorbed into the blood on passing through the tubules, the rate of passage of the 99mtc.DTPA through the kidneys becomes ameasure of renal clearance. Binding sites in the renal tubules include thiol and disulfide moieties of various proteins (61), characteristics of the static kidney imagers include high binding site affinities, plasma

22

protein binding, and low liver uptakes (62), there are many complexes compound labeled with ^{99m}TC used as active transport for renal secretion process (63) such as N, N-bis (mercapto acebtmido)-ethylediamine (DADS) and o-iodo hippuric acid.

1.3.4 liver maging

The use of 99mtrc-labelled compound in hepatobiliay imaging was introduced in 1972 with the use of tc-penicillamine and then awide variety of 99m tc-complexes have been designed for this purpose (64). In designing any labeled compound to image bepatobilary function, one must attempt to minimize excretion by the kidneys and maximize extraction by the liver. The physical properties determining the favored excretory pathway of an agent are its size, charge, protein binding and functional group hydrophobicity, the more lipophilic species tend to be excreted by the liver and the hydrophilic species by the kidneys (65).

Two general types of ligands have been combined witb technetium to form hepatobiliary imagng agents, these include the iminodiacetic acid complexes, and the pyridoxylideneaminate complexes (66,67). The latter are composed of Schiff basses to which various hydrophobic amino acids are attached, these complexes are believed to have 99mtc

23

in the IIIoxidation state, best owing a (-1) charge on the complexes.

This means that the uptake in hepatocytes is determined primarily by the anionic active transport process and by the way the complexes fit into the carrier proteins of that system (68).

1.3.5 heart imaging:

^{99m}TC -complexes may become a major competitor of 201TI. ^{99}IC is preferred because o its shorter half-life, six hours compared to 72 hours for the 201TI, lower cost, and greater availability. Although group I cations (K_{+1}, CS_{+1} and R_{b+}) accumulate in normal myocardium through the action of the Na+/K+ ATPase system, so radioactive isotopes of these cations can be used for heart imaging. Awide variety of other cations including TI, also accumulate in normal heart tissue, however, not through this enzyme system. Instead they are beleived to bind to relatively nonselective recpetors which appear to recobnize a variety of positively charged speciese. This has been the basis for the development of an entire group of potential technetium based heart-imaging agents (69,70).

Many authors have puplished th use of ^{99m}TC -labelled compounds in heart imaging agents (71-75). Because the 201TI and ^{99m}Tc isonitriles complexes will only reveal an absence of uptake in damaged heart tissue, localization of myocardial infarctions with these agents is difficult so ^{99m}Tc-complexes which accumulates specifically in the infarction tissue is necessary to quantity heart damage (76).

A number of 99mTc bone imaging agents have been found to localize in infaracted myocardium, most notably 99mtc-pyrophosphate was localized in damaged tissue producing a hot-spot rather than a cold-spot image of the infarct (77), it is agued that the localization is the result of irreversible deposition of calcium in the mitochondria due to the combination of cell membrane damage plus residual coronary blod flow to the damaged area (78). Other complexes such as ^{99m}tc-MDP, ^{99}tc-HMDP and ^{99m}tc-HEDP were studied and gave good damaged-to-normal heart concentration rations (79). Red blood cells and human serum albumin labeled with ^{99m}tc were also used to obtain perfusion images of the myocardium at the capillary level (80,81).

1.3.6 bone imaging:

Many radionuclides have been used in the investigation of bone metabolism both in animals and in human, include, phosphorous ^{32}P, calcium, ^{40}Ca, strontium, ^{87m}Sr, and barium, ^{137m}Ba. (82-85). The production of ^{99m}Tc-labelled phosphorous complexes has led to adistinct improvement in bone scintigraphy largely due to the lower energy of the gamma-ray and the greator radioactivity administered as compared to the previously used radionuclides (86), several abnormal patterns of bone scintigrams with ^{99m}Tc-labelled phosphorous complexes have been reported in patients with metabolic bone diseases (87,88).

1.4. ^{99}TC-PHOSPHATE COMPLEXES AS BONE SCANNING AGENTS.

Various chelating phosphate compounds labeled with reduced 99mTC have been proposed for bone imaging, these include short and long chain polyphosphates (89), pyrophosphate (90,91), and various diphosphonates, all these labelled compounds proved to be more or less effective bone imaging agents (92-94). It was found that 99mTc bone imaging agents could be produced with polyphosphates and hydroxyethlidene diphosphonate (HEDP), was know to inhibit bone growth, thus its interaction with the hydroxyapatite mineralization process had been established (95, 96). A number of new bone seeking tracers have been developed to improved bone affinity and stability characteristics by chemical substitution of one or both hydrogen atom (s) of the methylene group of MDP, the relationships between chemical structure and skeletal uptake of phosphonic acids in which carboxy groups were interoduced (97).

Bull etal. (98) have studied the 99mTc-2,3-dicarboxy propane-1. 1-diphosphonic acid (^{99m}Tc-DPD), they claimed that this compound has a good stability and compared it with ^{99m}Tc-MDP, 2hours after tracer injection. Dalrich and his coworkers

(99) have studied the comparision of bone imaging with ^{99m}Tc-DPD and ^{99m}Tc-MDP, their results comparing the bone to soft tissue ratios, showed that the difference between these agents were very small. The quality of bone image obtained depends upon the nature of the diphosphonate (100,101), this study as result of two integral parts:

1- comparative radioanalytical determinations and in vivo biokinetic.

Properties of the ^{99m}Tc-MDP, ^{99m}TC-EHDP and 99mTc-DPD bone seeking agents.

2- Clinical comparison of the imaging characteristics or ^{99m}Tc-MDP and. Te-DPD.

Wang etal. (102,103) evalued several MDP analogus in eats, bydroxymethane diphosphonate (HMDP) (104, 105), 2, 3-dicarboxypropane-1, diphosphonate (DPD) (106) have been studied, the authors suggested that the last two compounds are superior to MDP by virtue of improved uptake in normal bone. Domstad etal. (107) obtained comparable bone images and similar average lesion/normal bone ratios with MDP and HMDP in two groups or patients. In another study involving 20 patient and 10 normal volumteers (108), there were no appreciable differences between MDP and HMDP with regard to blood level, bone to background ratio or appearance of the skeleton. It was suspected that the ^{99m}Tc-DP accumulate on or incorporated within the actively growing bydroxyapitie (HA) crystals.

Because ^{9m}Tc-DP accumulates in regions of new bone formation the agents are used to image skeletal condition, involving accelerated bone turnover, such as the remodeling of bone break or in the compenstotory new bone response that accompanies acancerous osteolytic lesion (93, 109). Visualization of new growing bone is the most unique and important use of ^{99m}Tc-bobe imaging agents in this regard, studies have been conducted to determine which ^{99m}Tc-DP have the highest uptake in new growing bone (110). The back bone of the diphosphonate ligands used in nuclear medicine and its related compound shown in fig 1 (1,10).

Parent molecute

methylene diphosphonate (MDP)

Pyrophosphate(PP)

ethane-1-hydroxy -1,1-
Diphosphonate (EHDP)

hydroxymethane
Diphosphonate (HMDP)

N-(methylamino) methylene
Diphosphonate (NMMDP)

N,N-dimethylamino methylene
Diphosphonate (DMAD)

3-amino-1-
hydroxy propane -1,1-
Diphosphonate (APD)

2,3- dicarboxy propane -1,1-
Diphosphonate (DPD)

Fig (1,10): structural formula of diphosphonate and pyrophosphate (110).

Empirical studies with ^{99m}Tc-polyphosphate have demonstrated that the longer chain length of the polyphosphate (n=2 to n=30) the lower the uptake of the ^{99m}Tc-complex in bone (111-113), fig (1.11) show the parent molecule of these compounds.

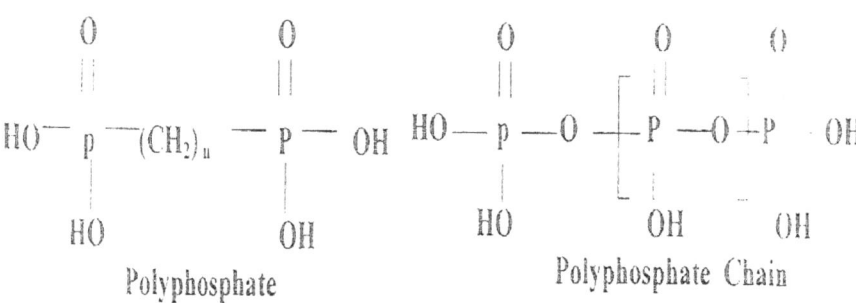

Polyphosphate   Polyphosphate Chain

Fig(1.11):Parent molecule of polyphosphate.

Similar studies with several polymethylene diphosphonate reveal that the samaller the diphosphonate ligand, the higher the uptake in bone and the lower the uptake in muscle and blood (114, 115). There are several studies which show that the diphosphonate compounds have excellent physical and chemical properties as bone scanning agents (116). They provide highly reproducible bone scane despite variations in Tc-presentation, labeling and injection procedures (108), the variation in temperature and pH have minimal effect on stability of the labelledosteodystrophy show an increased skeletal uptake of 99mTc-laelled compounds (118).

Zimmer etal. (119) have suggested that enzymes such as alkaline phosphate complexing with diphosphnate may explain uptake of tracer on bone surfaces, this eems unlikely in paget's disease for example high this enzyme there would be considerable delay in blood clearance of DP and this does not occur (120).

1.4.1 the natue of ^{99m}Tc-diphosphonate bone scanning agents:

^{99m}Tc-diphosphonate are mixture of many compounds that may differ in the valency of Tc, the number of DP-ligands, the nature and steric position of other ligands and the degree of polymerization, the composition of reaction mixture is governed partly by thermodynamic and partly kinetics (121). The properties of Tc-bone seeking labelled compounds, the valence of tc, the size of the complex ions, their charge and molecular composition have been studied (122-127). 99mTc-labelled compounds appear to give less bone uptake when Cr (II), Mo (III) and. W (III) were used as reducing agents corresponding with that prepared with Sn (II) (128-130), other authors had studied the using of other reducing agents such as Hg-electrode at 1.3v vs. SCE at Ph 7.0 (131), and NaBH$_4$ (132, 133).

1.4.2 ^{99m}Tc-MDP as bone scanning:

Since its introduction ^{99m}Tc-MDP has become the most common agent for imaging the skeleton (134). Mele and his coworkers (135) suggest that MDP has a higher bone uptake and alower sot-tissue retention in comparison with other diphosphonate labelled compounds the data presented by pauwels etal (136) showed that the new bone seeking agents DPD and HDP do not possess clinical advantages over MDP to detect of skeletal metastases. The lesion to normal bone ratio was significantly higher for MDP than for DPD, other have studied the value of local ^{99m}Tc-MDP bone to soft tissue uptake ratio in osteoporosis before and after floride therapy (137). Tuomo (138) was studied the use of ^{99m}Tc-MDP for sacroiliac seintigraphy, he suggested that MDP was the agent of choice for imaing sacroiliac joints. There are other studies of the clinical application of ^{99m}Tc-MDP in unclear a placation (139-143).

The properties of an ideal bone imaging agent may differ according to the clinical application (144-146):

1- to delineate benign or malignant focal lesions, which is the most frequent indication a high ratio of lesion-to-normal bone uptake, at the same time there must be sufficient activity in normal bone for accurate localization of lesions, balanced against low background activity in soft tissues such as the muscles and major viscera (liver, spleen, kidneys and lungs).

This is chieved by rapid clearance of plasma activity without diffusion into the red blood cells, which in turn requires a high renal extraction efficiency. Fortunately, MDP do not undergo gastrointestinal or biliary exeretion so that gastrointestinal activity dos not obscure the lumbar spine or pelvis (145).

2- To   as a vascular necrosis, both normal uptake and the bone-to-soft tissue ratio must be high. For quantitation of skeletal activity at 24 hours in patients with generalized bone disease, Fogelman (144) prefers ethane -1-hydroxy-1, 1-diphosphonate (EHDP) because of its lower overlap between normal and abnormal bone uptake than with other diphosphonates.

1.5 COMPETITIVE – BINDING STUDIES

In the last 1960's it has become possible to quantify great variety of organic substances by means of competitive protein-binding techniques using radionuclide labelled substat. These have offered so many advantages over the others and have become so widespread in their applications (147). These studies are based on the non-covalet reverable binding of ligand to aspecific binding protein, according to the following general reaction:

Ligand + binding protein $\rightarrow$ binding protein –ligand……..(1)

Examples of specific binding protein are antibodies coricosteroed binding globuline (CBG), estrogen receptors, thyroglobulin (TBG) and others. These proteins are characterized by their ability to bind ligands (varied antigens, cortisol, corticosterone, estrogen, vitamin B12....etc) with high specificity and affinity. The competitive-binding assay can be imaged as the addition of increasing amount of unlabelled ligand to reaction mixtures containing known constant amounts of labelled ligand which compelte for the binding site of specific inding protein (148).

$$Ab + L \rightarrow Ab{:}L \ldots\ldots\ldots\ldots\ldots\ldots..2$$

$$L^* + Ab \rightarrow Ab{:}\ L \ldots\ldots\ldots\ldots\ldots 3$$

L^* = labelled ligand

Ab=antibody

If the conditions are selected correctly, then over a certain dose range of non radioactive will be bound to the binding protein and does response curve in term of non radioactive added and either bound to the binding protein or existing free unbound solution may be dr wn (148). Common types of markers used to labell ligands include radioisotopes, enzymes, and fluorphores. These can be used both homogenous and hetergenous competitive binding assays. The sensitivity of binding reaction assay is function of the affinity of the binding protein for its ligand. The specificity of binding protein for its ligand is measured by its abitity to bind only the ligand and not other substances. Avarious assay techniques using the same basic principles of competive binding assays include (147, 149-152):

1- readioimmuno assay, which have the ligand and constant amount of radioactively labelled ligand compete for alimited number of antibody binding sites. Redioimmuno assay is applicable to the measurement of both low-molecular weight and high molecular weight ligands.

2- Enzyme-linked immunosorbent assay (ELISA):

Are heterogenous nonisotopie assays that usually have an antibody immobilized onto a solid support and the ligand labelled with the enzyme.

3- Homogneous enzyme immuno assay: the binding of antibody to the enzyme-labelled ligand changes the enzymatic activity of the labell so that antibody – bound enzyme can be distinguished from unbound labelled ligand.

4- Substrate – labelled flurescance immno assay:

This assay is based on a lebel that is a flurogenic enzyme substrate. When the label is hydrolyzed by aspecific enzyme (β-galactosidase) it yields afluorescent product.

5- Florescence polarization immunoassay : is based on the amount of polarized fluorescent light detected when the fluorophore label is excited with polarized light.

6- Apoenzyme reactivation immunoassay system (ARIS):

Has bee applied to dry reagent strip tests for analysis of therapeutic drugs such as thophylline,phenytouin.

1.5.1 protein labeling with ^{99}Tc and its complexes

For the clinical applications, ^{99m}Tc or its labelled compound are injected into the blood stream, it may bind reversibly and irreversibly to the blood protein, to investigate protein bnding, the protein bound ^{99m}Tc diphosphonate complexes must be separated from the free ^{99m}Tc-DP complexes either by precipitaton of protein with ammonium sulphate, trichoroacetic acid (TAC) (153, 154), gel chromatography (155, 156), ultrafilteration dialysis methods (157). The sum of reversibly and irreversibly bound ^{99m}Tc-DP can be observed when precipitaton with ammonium sulphate or ultrafilterration is used, in TCA method the values were high because of the decomposition of the ^{99m}Tc-DP complexes in th strongly acid solution and subsequent binding of the ^{99m}Tc to the denatured proteins. Reversibly bound protein ^{99m}Tc-DP complex will dissociate during chromatography only the Tc that is irreversibly bound to protein is observed (156, 157).

Interaction of aseries of ^{99m}Tc-labelled compounds with human blood proteins was investigated from two aspects: total protein binding and specificity of binding to certain classes of protein. The total protein binding of human sera with thireen ^{99m}Tc-labelled compound after in vitro labeling was determine by a precipitation method, dialysis and ultrafiltration (158). Many auther have studied total protein binding or binding with HSA as a model (159-166). The in vivo and in vitro study of the same complexes mentiond above have been done to calculate the selective binding to individual protein classes using agarose gel electrophoresis (167, 168), others have studied the total protein binding or biding with HSA (167, 168). Richard etal. (169) have investigated the uptake of ^{99m}Tc-MDP in the metaphysis and shaft of the rat femur as affected by hypophysectomy and hormonal replacement with growth hormone and thyroxine.

In vitro binding of ^{99m}TcO4 and its lablled compounds (gluconate and thiolat) of the structure (TcOL2)-1 and 99mTc-HSA have been investigated at very low protein saturation using equilibrium dialvsis and gel filteration methods (170). The stability of ^{99m}Tc-phosphorous compounds in olasma both in vivo and in vitro was studied using paper chromatographic technique as analytical tool (171), the result indicate that the amount of 99mTc activity found both at the origin and Rf range of ^{99m}TcO4 for in vitro or control, there for it is suggested that ^{99m}Tc-phosphorous labelled compounds are stable n vivo and neither oxidation nor hydrolysis of these bone imaging agents occurs in the blood. Albumin and red blood cells were labelled also with ^{99m}Tc and used for clinical applications (172-174).

1.5.2 some applications of labelled protein with 99mTc in nuclear medicine

Protein labelled with 99mTc have vry important applications in diagnostic nuclear medicine (175, 176). There are many parameters, such as labeling efficiency, stability of labelled attachment and retained biological behavior, e,g, immnoreactivity of monoclonal antibodies after radiolabelling must be studied carfully. Radiolabelled monocleonal atibodies (MoAbs) have great importance in diagnostic nuclear medicine because of thir highly specific targeting, tese antibodies hold considerable promises for the detection of primary and metastatic tumour sites (177) and in imaging of some benign conditions, e.g. for the assessment of damaged tissue in acute myocardial infarction or inflammatory lesions (178, 179). Some methods have been described for protein labeling with ^{99m}Tc and its application in unclear medicine (180-184). Maritta P., etal. (185) studied the optimization of derivtization of monoclonal antibodies and thier fragments intended for use in redioimaging or rado immunotherapy of prostatic cancer (158). Several ^{99m}Tc-labelled compound such as ^{99m}Tc-dimercaptosucciic acid (186), ^{99m}Tc-ethylenediamine-N, N-diaceltic acid and ^{99m}Tc-amino acids (187) are known to show high uptake in tumour high uptake of 99mTc-labelled DL-homocysteine in eeral tumours in vivo, and further investigation of the chemical properties have been studied (188, 189).

The aim of this work include the following:

1- development a method for albumin separation, purification and characterization from normal human blood. This method must be established for mass production of this protein for clinical uses and applications.

2- Characterization of the receptor or binding protein in human blood that carry the ^{99m}Tc-MDP to its target organ, bone or skelection, for diagnostic purposes.

3- Study some of the physicochemical proparties of ^{99m}Tc-MDP complexes with HSA , and bone homogenate, and then to estimate the effective parameters such as, the maximum binding (Bmax) of ^{99m}Tc-MDP with HSA and bone.

4- To established amethod for bone protein separation and then to study the binding parameters of this protein with ^{99m}Tc-MDP.

5- Kinestic and thermodynamic studies on the binding of ^{99m}Tc-MDP with HSA and bone homogenate, through determination of maximum binding capacities (Bmax) affinity constant (Ka), the parameter of equilibrium rections, apparent values of standard (ΔG_0, ΔH_0, ΔS_0) using van't hoff polt of the binding constants transition state thermodynamic parameters of the formation of ^{99m}Tc-MDP-HSA complex using Arrhenius plots, the rate constants of association and dissocation (K_{eq}) and the values of hill coefficient.

General knowledge

Isotopes in clinical chemistry:

The isotopic properties will make the labeled compound more easily identifiable. For example, the radiodine-lablled thyroxine molecules can be identified and quantified easily by virtue of their radioactivity.

The use of isotopes, both stable and radioactive, has provided great body of information in the medical science. Stable isotopes are non radioactive and are suitable for use as tracers in humans, especially infants children and pregnant women, stable isotopes have also been used in the quantitative analysis of various substances in recent years.

Radioactivity measurments depends on the ability of radionuclides to produce ionized or excited atoms within the detector. Two basic types of radiation detectors are in common use : gas ionization and scintillation. Radioisotopes allow the detection of minute quantities and differentiate physically between substances.

The use of radioactive isotopes in biochemistry and clinical chemistry has provided us with a wealth of information about biological processes, that offers such as adiverse range of applications, using enzyme assays, biochemical pathways of synthesis and degradation, analysis of biomolecules, measurements of antibodies, binding and transport studies.

The use of radionuclide in nuclear medicine began when Frederick proescher published the paper entitled the use of radium for therapy of various diseases. Early experimental and diagnostic applications were performed with naturally occurring radionuclides, then the radioisotope with physical short half lives have become increasingly popular for imaging applications.

The first commercially available radioisotope generator was the 134Ie-132I, (5) several other generators (such as ^{99}Mo-^{99m}Tc, ^{68}Ga, ^{113}Sn-^{113}In, ^{87}Y-^{87M}Sr---etc,) subsequently evolved (6-9). These generators must meet certain physical basic criteria to be useful. It should be simple and converient to operate, its radiation must be adequately shielded_____ yield adaughter product of high purity in terms of both radioaetivity and stable contaminants during every elution throughout the life of the generator, the product should be in achemical form suitable for use with aminimum of additional chemical or physical manipulation, lastly the radioactive yield of the daughter product during each elution should be high (10, 11).

Labeled compounds either be used in biochemical research or for routine medical diagnosis were carried out in vivo for medical diagnosis such as those labeled with gamma emitting isotopes to permit detection external to the patient, (12) but those labeled with beta-emitting isotopes such as: C, H, S, and P were principally used in biochemical research (13).

There are various methods which were used for preparing labeled compounds such as of the following:

(1) isotope exchange reactions, in which one or more atoms in the molecule, exchange with atoms of the same element and of different mass, these atoms may be radioactive or stable isotopes, according to the follwing:

$$AX^*+BX-BX^*+AX$$

The comound BX under certain reaction conditions will exchange its X atoms (s) with the compound AX^* where X^* atom (s) is an isotopic form of the element X, awide range of compounds labeled with different stable or radioactive isotopes are prepared by exchange methods, which have the advantage that they can normally be carried out on a small chemical scale, an example is the preparation of urea- C, (14-15).

$$CO(NH_2)2+14CO_2-CO(NH_2)2+CO$$

(2) chemical synthesis: involves the construction of complex molecules from simple isotopically labeled intermediates, yields are usually expere___ as a percentage radiochemical yield:

%radiochemical yield = Total radionactivity in product x100

Total radionactivity in substrate

For example, the preparation of earboxyl-labelled fatty acids by reation with the corresponding Grignard reagent or acetic anhydride-14°C, steroids-14°C and amino acid-14C (16-19)

(3)   biochemical methods : these include different procedures such as enzymatic synthesis which is very similar to chemical synthesis in that such a conversion usually occurs without any change in the specificity of the labeling or the molar specific activity (16). Total biosynthetic methods are normally of value only when microorganisms are employed, but the production of uniformly labeled carbohydrates by photosynthesis in detached leaves is an exception to this (17,18).

(4)   Recoil labeling (19, 20): this method depend on the ability of recoil atom produced in a nuclear reaction to form a stable bond with an organie (or an inorganic) compound. For example, if an organic compound is mixed with a lithium carbonate or chloride and irradiated in anuclear reactor at fixed neutron flux, tritium compounds are produced by the recoiling "tritond" from the nuclear reaction 6Li (n,) 3H.

One pure radioisotope or in labeled compounds is technetium-^{99m}Tc, which have a short half-life, about six hours, with a predominate single photon gama emissiom having an energy of 140 kev (21). ^{99m}Tc-labelled compounds are diagnostic imaging agents used in the field of nuclear medicine to visualize tissue anatomical structures and metabolic disorders. After intravenous administration ^{99m}Tc or its labeled compound localized in specific target organ or tissue, can then be imaged using stable instrument (22).

1.2 TECHNETIUM CHEMISTRY

Technetium is not a naturally abundant element, some of its properties were produced by Mendeleev in 1869, who called it ekamanganese and gave it the symbol (EM) (23). After world war II, Perrier and segre gave element 43 the name technetium as the first artiticial element (24).

Te chemistry is similar to its neigh bouring elements manganese and rhenium, a comprehensive review on tc-chemistry was published by deutch et al (25), some of physical properties of tc are shown in table (1.1).

Table (1.1): some of tc physical properties

Property	Value
Melting point	$2250 \pm 50 \, ^{\circ}C$
Density	$11.5 g/cm^3$
Atomic weight	98.913
Ionization potential	7.28 ev
Entropy of crystallization	7.4 ± 0.2 e.u.
Critical temperature or super conducting	7.7 kelven
Stable electronic state	4s 4p 4d 5s

To give rise to multiple oxidation states and forms coordination complexes with avariety of inorganic and organic ligands (26). The chemistry of tc im its I-V oxidation states was surveyed by davison and jones, many of the thermodynamically stable tc-complexes have oxygen bound to it like TcO_4, TcO_2-2H2O, Tc-O-ligand (27-29). Tc V and IV complexes are known to have the ligands coordinated to the tc alone, i-e tc Ln, Tc_2Ln---etc, the polynuclear formation of tc species is usually minimized by keeping the tc-concentration as low as possible, to prevent the formation of Ic complexes with more than one oxidation state, efforare made to control the reducing agent and the reaction conditionsfig (1.1) show some of tc-complexes at different oxidation state (30)

1.2.1 PRODUCTION OF 99MTC

^{99m}Tc is usually produced from agenerator system as aresult of the decay of molybdenum ^{99}Mo according to the follwing equation:

Generators have been developed to take the advantage of this property and make ^{99m}Tc widely available in unclear medicine laboratories (31), the generator containing ^{99}Mo as sodium molybdate adsorbed on to an aluminium oxide column shown in fig (1.2), ^{99m} tc is continuously formed by the decay of ^{99}Mo, elution of the column with isotonic saline yieded solution of pertechnetate which is chemically stable, sterile, pyrogen free and almost molybdenum and aluminium free (32,33). Generators can either be eluted by negative pressure, where there is attore of saline at the input to the column and an evacuated vial is placed over the outlet, or by positive pressure, where a quantity of saline is pushed through the column and the eluate collected in sterile vial with needle attached.

^{99}Mo is available from one of two soueither from neutron bombardment of 98in reactors (34), or from chemical sepaution of the fission products of uranium-(235), (35) in this case all Mo is in the form of ^{99}Mo and the column itself can be made more efficient and eluted with a small valume of saline, thus a higher specific activity eluted can be obtained which is usefull in various areas of clinical application (36).

1.2.2 PRINCIPLES OF LABELLING WITH TECHNETIUM:

The labeling of biologically important molecules with tc means the introduction of a foreign element. Though the exact nature of the chemical bonding of tc is still controversial, we can draw some important general conclusions from the viewpoint of periodic relationships (37).

Tc is amember of group VII B of the periodic table of the elements, thus belonging to the transition elements. Transition elements are those having partly filled (d) or (f) shells. Tc as an elements of the second series has partly filled 4d shells. The seven electrons in tc (beyond the noble gas configuration) are easily stripped to yield tc (VII) ((generator eluate)) as the stable compound at the oxidation state +7 is the staring material for preparation of tc-labelled compounds (38,39).

The principle of labeling has been shown to be complex formation (40-43). Tc in complexes is surrounded by anions or neutral molecules (lighands). Mono-dentate ligands such as (F, CI, CN….) donate only one electron pair to the tc atom, and its complexes with tc are not stable in neutral aqueous solution. Multidantate ligands (chelate ligands) are suitable substances for labeling with tc, as shown in table (1.2). complex formation occurs for compounds possessing functional groups such as hydroxyl, carboxyl, amino, phosphate…. Etc. in appropriate molecular arrangement. Hence, using current labeling procedures, hydrophilic substances that contain chelate moieties are the predominat source of tc-labelled compound. This implies preferable application of ionized biochemical and drugs (eg. Hydroxycarboxylates, mercaptocarboxylates, phosphate compounds….etc.) instead of pure lipophilic substance.

Table (1.2) : some typical substances used for the preparation of ^{99m}Tc labeled compounds.

Substances	Functional groups
Citrate	OH, COOH
Gluconate	OH, COOH
Glucoheptonate	OH, COOH
Sugars	OH
DTPA	COOH, IDA
Dimercaptosuccinate	SH, COOH
Mercaptoisobutyrate	SH, COOH
Penicillamine	SH,NH2, COOH
EHDP	OH, PO3H
MDP	PO3H
6-mercaptopurine	SH, arom-N

The binding of a chelating group and some of biological molecules to tc may be as in fig (1.3).

Initial applications of this approach have been reported to proteins and fatty acids (44,45). The complex of MDP with. Tc proved to be polymeric with technetium centres bridged by MDP and OH ligands (46) as shown in fig (1.4).

A general scheme in fig (1.5) show the reactions which have to be considered in the preparation of ^{99m}Tc-labelled compound.

1.2.3 methods of detection:

^{99m}tc either be administrated to a patient as sodium pertechnetate or it may be labeled with a range of compounds with a variety of useful biological distributions. The administered activity can be recorded with appropriate radiation detectors such as scanners, gamma cameras, whole nuclear medicine basically acts as atransducer which transforms incoming radiation into visible light (47) as in fig (1.6).

The detection of radioactivity is carried out by one of the three following methods:

1- detecting areas of increased concentration of the radioistop tracer within an area of relative homogeneous distribution of the labeled complex (hot spot imaging) as seen in brain tumours, bone metastases and myocardial infarction (48,49). Fig (1.7) show one these cases.

2- Detecting areas of reduced concentration of the radioactive tracer within a uniform radioactive organ (clod spot imaging) as in liver tumours, renal and thyroid cysts, (50, 51) fig (1.8) show one of these cases.

3- Monitoring the arrival and disappearance of the radioactivity over an area of interest ((time activity curves)) over the kidneys as in renography, fig (1.9) the brain as in cer bral perfusion studies, or the heart as in left ventricular volume curves.

1.3. ^{99m} TC-APPLICATION IN NUCLEAR MEDICINE

The following are some applications of ^{99m}tc and its labeled compounds in unclear nedicine.

1.3.1 thyroid imaging:

The trapping of ^{99m}tc as sodium pertechnetate by thyroid is useful for assessing both function and its anatomy of the gland (52), although thyroid gland requires iodide ion for the production of thyroxine and triodothyronine the iodide ions are transported across the membranes of the epithelial cells in the thyroid follicles by means of an active transport process, but the radius of iodide is comparable to that of pertechnetate and each of the ions has asingle negative charge then they have asimilar charge densities, so that $^{99m}TcO_4$ is taken up readily by thyroid cells, even though iodine has several gamma-energies, so $^{99m}tco_4$ is preferred (29).

1.3.2 brain imaging:

It is limited to the detection of ruptures of tumours and vascular lesions that impair the function of the blood brain barrier which is normally impermcable to the highly water-soluble ^{99m}tco4 (53). The rate at which substances penetrate brain tissue through the blood-brain barrier is inversely related to their size and directly related to their lipid solubility (54), therefore attempts have been made to design small tc-complexes with hydrophobic ligands such as bis-aminorthanethiol, propylene amine oxime (55). Each of these agents readily crosses the blood brain barrier but subsequently clears the brain tissue in a matter of minutes due to the lack of affinity for any particular receptor sites to these agents (56,57).

1.3.3 kidney imaging:

Nearly all 99mtc-labelled compounds will be excreted by the kidneys and eliminated in the urine, because of the kidneys are the principle organ responsible for the excration of water-soluble substances from the body the functional unit of the kidney is called the nephron, it is composed of a filtering apparatus referred to as the glomerulus, which is encapsulated in

Purification and spectroscopic characterization of human serum albumin (HSA)

SUMMARY

This chapter deals with the purification and characterization of human serum albumin (HSA), anew method of albumin purification from human blood was followed. The characterization was carried out through electrophoresis and spectroscope studies. Facters affecting the absorption have been atudied. The effect of solvent perturbation and pH perturbation were also studied, the results indicats that there are different effects of these solvents (such as ethanol, urea, DMSO, …etc) on the HSA spectrum. The pH titration of albumin show that about 30% of the tyrosyl residues are located on the surface of HSA molecules whereas 70% were buried interior the molectules.

INTERODUCTION

Albumin is a single polypeptide containing 584 residues with N-terminal asp and c-terminal leu. There is alarge number of glu, asp and lys residues which a counts for the high polarity and hence solubility of the protein, it contains no carbohydrate and the molecular weight of albumin is around 66300 (190).

The procedures of isolation of albumin from blood were dependent on the use of the high stability of albumin at various conditions, (191) where most of plasma proteins are denatured, precipitation with trichloracetic acid follwed by ethanol extraction (4), selective precipitation with dextran sulphate

(192), rianol (193), polyethyleneglycol (194) may be used for isolation. However, these methods are associated with the problems of removal of the precipitating agents (192-194), there are several methods that deals with the separation of albumin such as those of ion exchange chromatography (195) and affinity chromatography (196). Whereas the first method used for albumin separation was depended on the low temperature-alcohol (197), the disadvantage of this method is related to the low yield (60%). The best spectroscopic methods for characterization of albumin are the solvent perturbation techniques (198). In the solvent perturbation method of probing the surface of protein molecules, advantage is taken from the fact that the spectra of chromophoric residues coming freely in contact with the solvent are sensitive to changes in the physical properties of the solvent, such as refractive index, dielectric constant, and solvent-solute interactions, in the immediate vicinity of the chromophores (199). There are several studies on the application of solvent perturbation technique of difference spectroscope such as those related to studying the location of chromophoric side chains in gloubular proteins (milk proteins, α-lacta albumin, β-locatoglobulin, bovine serum albumin…etc) dissolved in aquecous media (198-201). This chapter deals with the characterization of isolated albumin and then with the extension of this solvent perturbation technique of difference spectroscopy to the study of the properties of purified (HSA) in aqueous solvents.

2.1 INSTRUMENTS AND CHEMICALS USED

2.1.1 instruments used:

1- cooling centrifuge model MSE, mistral, 3000i with maximum speed of 5000 rpm, made in orion research incorporated camberdge U.K.

2- cooling system with mixer, thermocouple, prestatic pump- and temperature control unit, manufactured in Iraqi atomic energy commission specialist for this perpose.

3- orion-pH meter.

4-elecrophoresis system, Sartorius, multiphor system.

5- hitashi U-2000 spectrophotometer.

2.1.2. chemicals:

All common laboratory chemicals and reagents used in this chapter were of analar grade, obtained from fluka company, Switzerland (NaH_2PO_4, NaH_2PO_4, NaCL, KCl, $CaCl_2$ and $MgCl_2$), ethanol, acetic acid, sodium acetate, sodium carbonate and sodium bicarbonate, from BDH, limited pool U.K, polyethylene glycol (PEG-4000) from LKB, Switzerland, sephadex, from pharmacia fine chemicals, Switzerland, standard human serum albumin, albumin novo nordisk, DK 2880 Bagsvaer, denmark.

2.1.3 buffers:

All buffer solutions were prepared by dissolving the appropriate amount of salts in distilled water and the required pH was adjusted with pH meter. The buffers required were, phosphate buffer ($Na_2HPO_412H_2O$ with NaH_2PO_4) acetate buffer (acetic acid with sodium acetate) and carbonate buffer (sodium carbonate with bicarbonate).

2.2 ALBUMIN PURIFICATION

A modified method of HSA purification was used in this chapter. The modification depends on the use of polyethylene glyecol (PFG-4000) to separate fibrinogen, lipoprotein and immunoglobulin, then ethanol was used to remove any tracer of other proteins remaining with albumin. The procedure was carried out according to the following steps:-

1- the human blood was collected from national center for blood transfusion its pH was adjusted to 7.2 using acetate buffer, then it was centrifuged at-4c and 3600 rpm for 25 minutes to remove any coagulant particles from plasma, the plasma was separated and its volume was measured.

2- separation of albumin is commenced by precipitation with 16% w/v polyethylene glycol-4000 to avoid coprecipitation of albumin with immunoglobulin. In this step nearly all high molecular weight material (such as fibrinogen, β-lipoprotein…etc) were removed. The addition of PEG solution was carried out very slowly at-5c with continuous stirring for one hour, then the mixture was centrifuged at 3600 rpm and-5°c, the supernatant was collected, its pH was adjusted to 4.8 using acetate buffer or carbonate buffer solution.

3- a second precipitation step using 25% w/v PEG-4000 was carried out to the supernatant collected in step 2, the required amount of PEG was added very slowly with continuous stirring at-5c (ethanol-water cooling system), the pH must be adjusted to 4.8. the precipitated albumin then was centrifuged at 3600 rpm and -5c, the precipitate must washed several times with the same buffer at 0c to remove any tracer of PEG remaining as contamining with albumin. The crude albumin then was dissolved in phosphate buffer-saline solution.

4- the pH of the solution obtained from step 3 was adjusted to 5.2 using carbonate buffer, then ethanol 95% was added dropewise with continuous stirring in a cooled system (-5°c) to get final concentration of ethanol equal to that of 40% v/v, stirring must be continued for another one hour, then the mixture was centrifuged at-4c and 3600 rpm, the supernatant was collected (albumin solution), its volume was measured, the pH was then adjusted to 4.8 with carbonate buffer.

Another portion of 95% ethanol was added to the albumin solution obtained in step (4), to get final ethanol concentration of 10%, the addition was carried out stepwise at-5c with continuous stirring.

The precipitate (albumin) was separated by centrifugation at-5°c, the yield and the purity of albumin was more than 86% and 99% respectively.

The prepared albumin was lyophilized and then stored at 4c to be used in further experiments.

2.2.1 albumin determination:

Protein concentration was determined by the method of lowry et al (203) using HSA as the internal standard (fig2.1).

2.2.2 albumin characterization:

The lyophilized albumin was dissolved in physiological saline to get final concentration of 20% w/v as stock solution, the characterization of the albumin was carried out by:-

(a) electrophoresis :

Reagents: Sartorius cellulose acetate strips 5x12cm. corning barbital buffer pH 8.6, 5% v/v acetic acid, and micropipette.

Procedure:

Three spots of crude serum, standard HSA and purified HSA were placed on the cellulose acetate strips (approximately 5ml of each sample was used), the current used was about 12 mA, 4mA per strip) and 200 volts after about 75 minutes the power supply was switched off, the strips were removed from the tank and washing with 5% acetic acid then with water.

(b) U.V. absorption spectra of albumin:

100 µl of the albumin stock solution (1mg/ml) (the prepared albumin) was diluted to 50 ml with normal saline. At the same time 100µl of standard albumin (20% w/v) was diluted with 50ml normal saline. The U.V. absorption spectra of the prepared and standard albumin were measured in the area of 200-310 nm at pH7.0.

2.2.3 factors affecting the absorption properties of purified albumin:

2.2.3.1 pH effect:

The lyophilized HSA which was prepared was dissolved in phosphate buffer to get a concentration of 20% w/v as stock solution 100µl of this solution was diluted up to 50ml using the same buffer. The pH was adjusted by mixing 4ml of protein solution with required volume of dilutes solution of HCI or NaOH to prepare the sample at required pH then difference spectra were usually abtained. The aqueous solutions of amino acid tyrosine and phenylalanine were also prepared in distilled water at a concentration of $2x10^{-3}$ M&$2.5x10^{-3}$M respectively, in 50ml volumetric flask as stock solution. The required pH was adjusted by diluted solution of HCL and NaOH. The absorbance of each amino acid was measured at fixed pH region in the area of 200-300nm. The absorbance of albumin, tyrosine and phenylalanine were also measured at netural, acidic and basic pH.

2.2.3.2 effect of polarity:

The protein solutions were studied spectrophotometricelly by the addition of different solvents, such as, ethanol, urea, KCI, ethylene glycol, poly ethylene glycol, glycerol and dimethyl sulphoxide in a percent range of 10-20%, for example, ethanol: albumin solution was prepared as spectra of each sample was measured, at the same time samples of ethanol: tyrosine and ethanol: phenylalanine were prepared at the same percent and pH values were adjusted similarly.

The effect of increasing amount of ethylene glycol was studied using 5, 10, 20, 25 and 30% ethylene glycol: albumin mixture at pH 7.0, the absorbance spectra of each sample was measured after 30 minutes, at 200-300nm.

2.2.3.3 effect of some drugs on the albumin spectra:

Solutions of thyroxine (T4), cortisol and oleic acid were prepared in tri-N-butyl amine, each was mixed with albumin solution in a percentage of 1:4 (v/v), after 30 minutes the spectra of each sample was measured at the same area of wave length (200-300nm). The absorbance of solvents were subtracted by placing the solvent mixture in the reference cell and the protein mixture was put in the sample cell.

2.2.3.4 structural studies of albumin:

A series of albumin sample were prepared at pH range from 8 to 13, the maximum absorbance of each sample was measured at a wave length of 295nm, the absorbance of λ_{max} at each pH values were plotted vs corresponding pH. In parallel experiment a solution of pure tyrosine and phenylalanine at pH 12.6 were prepared and its absorbance spectra was measured similarly,

RESULTS AND DISCUSSION

Albumin purification:

Albumin is the most familiar and abundant of the plasma protens, it consists approximately 60% of the total serum protein and is synthesized almost exclusively by the liver, it is a small globular protein with high electrophoretic mobility which acts to maintain homeostasis in the body, its haemodynamic and transport functions by providing aprotein reserve (190, 202). The expired blood from national center for blood transfusion was used to purify the prepared albumin, in the first step of separation PEG-400 must be added at high concentration (50% stock solution) to prevent the contamination of albumin by gamma-globulin, the temperature used in the purification, the addition of PEG and pH adjustment of the serum are very important parameters, very good separation was achieved at-8 t0 50c, any decrease in pH value below 7.0 the fibrinogen and immunoglobulms were not separated quantitatively, and hence may be remained as a contaminant with albumin.

In step (3) of separation, pH must be adjusted to 4.8 to prevent either the loss of some albumin (i.e. decrease in the yield) or albumin contaminated with other lipoproteins (i.e. decrase the purity of albumin). Tracer amount of other proteins can be removed in step (4) and abumin was precipitated specifically in step (5) with ahigh purity and reproducibility.

Albumin characterization:

Electrophoresis:

Fig (2.2) show the electrophoresis profile for crude serum, purified and standard albumin, on cellulose paper electrophoresis. The bands corresponding to crude serum are multiple and referred to the different proteins molecules present in serum, while the albumin band both prepared and standard, show only one band at the end of negation the results medicate that the standard and prepared albumin are ident the purified albumin in this method has chemical purity identical to the standard albumin, and no any trace of contamination with other serum proteins are present.

Spectroscopic studies:

Fig (2.3) shows U.V. spectra (200-350nm) for two types of albumin molecules, standard and purified albumin from blood. The parameters usually measured are absorbance and the wavelength corresponding to a peack of maximum absorption (λmax) consist of multiple peaks, at 278.0nm, 238.8nm for purified HSA and 277.8nm, 238.8nm for standard albumin. As aresult, purified HSA have characteristic spectra and can be tyrosine, tryptophane and phenylalanine (204-209).

Factors affecting the absorption properties of purified HSA:

The absorption spectrum of HSA is primary determined by the chemical structure of the molecule. However, a large number of environmental factors produce detectable change in λmax and environmental factors consist of pH, the polarity of the solvent or neighbouring molecules, and the relative orientation of neighboring chromophores. It is precisely, these environmental factors effects provide the basis for the use of absorption spectroscopy in characterizing HSA. The general features of these environmental effects on the spectrum of the molecule are the following:

pH effect:

the pH of the solvent determines the ionization state of ionizable HSA. an example is shown fig (2.5 & 6) and table (2.2) which illustrates the effect of pH on tyrosine and phenylalanine spectra respectively. The data show that λmax are increased when phenolic OH is dissociated. Table (2.1) show an increase in λmax from 278.0nm to 295.0 nm when the pH of the HSA solution was increased from 7.0 to 12.8, while there is no significant change in λmax in the acidie region (when pH decreased from 7.0 to 1.6 ------be due to the slightly increasing in the energies of electronic trans of the aromatic rings from the formation of the electron-withdrawing ammonium groups (210). It is known that in the acidic region the phenolic OH group are not ionized, so there is no n-π* or π- π* transition. The same results were obtained with tyrosine where λmax was shifted from 274.8 at pH to 293.0nm at pH 12.6, but no any change in the λmax of phenylalanine both in acidic and basic region was obtained. In asimilar studies on tryptophane and o-methyl tyrosine, λmax were shifted towerd shorter wave lengths when the Ph was decreased from 11 to less than 7.0 (211, 212).

In the neutral and slightly acidic pH region, the native organization of the HSA is fairly compact and rigid, this has been suggested by the fact that neither pH nor ionic strength has any significant effect on the mean dimension of bovine serum albumin (BSA) calculated from viscositv and sedimentation data over afairly wide range of pH (213, 214).

Tanford and buzzell (215) have noted that the intrinse viscosity remains essentially constant between pH 4.3 and neutrality and that it is largely independent of the ionic strength in this pH region (214)

Effect of solvent polarity on HSA U.V. absorption:

Generally it is well known that the polar groups on the HSA, the value of λmax for π-π* transitions occurs at longer wave length when polar hydroxylic solvents (H_2O_2, alcohols) are used. Fig (2.7) and table (2.3), at high pH (12.6) shows the apperance of new λmax at 258nm which indiecate that the protein was defolded due to ethanol or achange in thesecondary and teriary structure of the protein that bring the phy-residues to the surface of the protein molecules, but there was no effect on the ma---- absorbance of HSA at pH 7.0 and 1.7, this indicate that there was ----- interaction or any change that happended between solvent and ------- moleules.

In the case of free tyrosine, table (2.3) and fig (2.7 and 2.8) shows shift of λmax toward shorter wave length at neutral (pH 7.0) and ---- region when 10% ethanol was used this may be due to ----- bonding formation between phenolic OH group of rosine with ethanol molecules or other interaction (i.e. hydrophobic, dipole-dpol, vander ---- interactions…..etc.) since these factors affect the n→π* transition (205), whereas there is no effect on phenylalanine spectrum fig (2.8), table (2.4) show the effect of increasing ethylene glyol concentration on the albumin (HSA) spectra (λmax), there was no significant effect at 5% ethylene glysol, but a shift towerd longer wave-length was obtained when the ethylene glycol concentrations were increased u 30%. These results indicat that, ethylene glycol effect the HSA structure causing an increase in λmax from 278nm to 291nm, this effect may be resulted from defolding of albumin molecule. The buried chromophoric groups may be a commodated equally well in hydrophobic area located between neighbroring helices or between hlical and nonhelical segments of the protein fold (216). The relatwely inert character of ethylene glycol has made it useful solvent for the study directed toward the elucidation of the sources of conformation stabil of proteins (217-219).

Table (2.5) and figs (2.9 and 2.10) show the effect of different solvents on albumin spectrum at pH 7.0. the data obtained show that there was no an effect of PEG and glycerol (the concentration of 20% and 50% on λmax at 278.2±0.2nm was obtained, which is similar to the HSA spectrum at neutral pH as shown in carlier experiments. These result indicate that there was no interaction between the solvents and HSA molecues at pH 7.0 since only the spectra of chromophores that have completely free access to the solvent will be shifted. Dioxan show a little decrease in the λmax that is from 278.2±0.2 to 277.7±0.1 and another absorption peak were appeared at λmax 232.8 and 236.4 at 20% and 50% dioxane, respectively. These two absorption peaks represent other chromohores than tyrosyl which as effected by dioxane structurally, hence the effect was expressed by the appearance of this chromophor on the surface of the HSA molecule, the new chromophor located near the tyrosyl residues is cearly seen.

In the case of DMSO (20%) two absorption peaks were obtained at λmax 300.0 and 276.2nm thus this solvent has agreat effect n the protain structure, λmax at 276.2 is related to tyrosyl residue was effected with optained at 300nm may be due to tryptophyl residues which is located at the surface of HSA molecules resulted from defolding of HSA, they absorption region may be due to π-π* transition, these results indicates that the salvation eergies of both excited and ground stated may be decreased by a polariazation of the solvent and the dipole moment of the excited state is greater than that of the ground state, hence greater stabilization of the excited state by salvation has occurred (220).

Table (2.6) show, the effect of 8M-urea on the HSA spectrum at pH7.0 and 3.8. at neutral pH no effect on the position of λmax was obtained, whereas there was a longer wave length shift at pH 3.8 and two absotrption peaks at 299.6 and 263.0nm, were obtained (fig 2.11). these observations indicate that urea have no effect on the protein structure at neutral pH even when the concentration was high up to 50% as in fig (2.12). there is only 1.6nm shift on going from 20% to 50% of urea concentration when 8M-ure was mixed with 0.03M-KCI at pH 6.2,the same shift as observed as in fig (2.11) 0.03M-KCI at neutral pH also show that therfomnce long wave shift (λmax=300.0nm), this means that the shift in the case of 8M urea and 0.03M KCI may be due to the effect of KCI but not to urea the long wave shift produced by urea appears to be lagely attributable to greater dispersive interaction, absence of significantly increased hvdrogen bonding in urea solution as compared to water alone is suggested by the fact that nearly equal spectral shift are obsevd by p-bromophenol and p-bromoanisole in 8M-urea (210).

The protein molecule is highly charged at the low pH region thus it expands considerably as electrostatic sereening due to extraneous salt is reduced, and urea produces an ppreciable isotropic swelling of the denaturation (12), or limited protelysis (222). These different spectra appear to be dependent on the changes in the polarity (dielectric constant), the plarizability (refractive index) (223), and the charge state of the immediate environment of the chromophoric residues and on the change in strong interactions such as hydrogen bonding (224). All of these are related, but hey change in acomplicated and largely unknown way with th changes in the conformation of the protein molecule.

Difference spectroscopy of HSA:

The λmax for HSA occurs in the same region of the spectrum but that there is often aslight dependence upon the HSA environment the dependence of spectra upon environment offers the possibility of determining structural information regarding the HSA. The changes produced by different environment are reatively small, it is more accurate and convenient to measure directly, the difference between the HSA in the two environment rather than make an absolute measurement of each one separately. This was achieved in a double beam spectrophotometer by placing one of the solutions in the eference compartement and the other in the sample compartement.

The spectrophotometer will then respond to the difference in absorption and the measurement of the variation of this difference with wave-length produces a difference spectrum. It is possible to change the environment in anumber of ways, but change in the solvent composition and pH were used in order to give the valuable information.

Fig (2.13) show the difference spectra of HSA vs a mixture of tyrosine $(2 \times 10^{-3} M)$ and phenylalanine $(2.5 \times 10^{-3} M)$, this experiment I based on the assumption that HSA containing 18 tyrosyl, 0.6 tryptophyl and 33 phenylalanyl resdues per one molecule of protein (199). From table (2.7) the λmax at pH 7.0 and 1.6 are nearly the same values and this value is not related to either tyrosine nor phenylalanine at the same pH region, but table (2.2), indicate that the λmax change is due to tryptophyl residues while at pH 12.6 the λmax absorbance is due to phenylalanine residues while means that there was achange in the protein structure in this pH ----- tryptophyl residues were buried interiorly. In the protein molecule. The disappearance of tyrosine absorbace (λmax=278nm) at pH 7.0 indiate that there was some tyrosyl residues on the surface of native HSA which was substractd when tyrosine solution was placed in the reference cell. The same conclusion may be applied to other pH values in the spectra.

Solvent perturbation studies:

One way in which the environment of HSA can be varied significantly is to alter the solvent composition. From the point of view of the protein te solvent is represented by all of the nonalbumin molecules if experiences around it. It would not be sensible to change the solvent completely from water to a non-aqueous system since denaturation would result. However, significant solvent effects can be induced by use of amixture of water and glycerol, ethylene glycol, dioxane and DMSO. Difference spectra for solvent perturbation found in HSA are shown in igure (2.15, 2.16) which sows that the difference in λmax and molarabsorption coefficient far to urea. PEG and DMSO exposure.

Perhaps the most application of the solvent perturbation techniques is in calculation the degree of exposure of certain amino acids on HSA surface. This is based on the premise that amino acids residues on the exterior of the HSA will be exposed to the solvents (urea, PEG, DMSO) and comtributed to adifferences in the spectra of HSA (figs, 2.15, 2.16).

Solvent perturbation difference spectra of HSA are shown in figs (2.15, b, 2.16, b) suggests that these difference spectra are due primarily to tyrosine and tryptophane. It is, of course, esse—ial to show that the solvent perturbation it self does not alter the HSA conformation. This is usually done by checking the linearity of the dependence of the perturbation (ΔE) with increasing concentration of the perturbant urea.

One of the main assumption of the solvent perturbation technique is that the perturbing solvent does not alter, in any serious manner, the conformation of the protein under investigation. Foster (225) has proposed amodel for HSA, the peptide chain is folded into four flat subunits, stacked one on the other with three interface between them the various isomerization reactions are envistaged as subunit separations. This model can well be used in discussing our solvent perturbation results, the tyrosyl residues must be located on one of the interfaces between the subunits and thus be inaccessible to bulky perturbing solvents (glycerol, ethylene glycol, poly ethylene glycol, dioxane ad DMSO).

Solvents alter the peak positions and intensities by changing the energy and probability of electronic. When both solute and solvent are polar, salvation energies are large in the ground state and there will form acage of oriented solvent molecules around each solute molecule, when transition occues the excited molecule will in general have assize and charge distribution different from those of the ground state, the solvent molecules of the cage will not have time to reorient themselves and will be in a state of strain, this will decrease the salvation energy of the excited state and in the absence of opposing effects, will produce a short wave shift (220). Two other effects must be considerd (226-28): (a) change in permanent dipolemoment during excitation i.e., the diol polarization effect. (b) Hyrogen bonding which will tend to produce either a short or long wave shift depending on the nature of the electronic transition and whether the solute is the hydrogen donor or hydrogen acceptor.

pH perturbation:

A great deal of information can be obtained by direct measurement of different spectra of HSA at different pH values. Figs (2.18, 2.19) show the difference spectrum of HSA due to the change pH. The curves represent absorption difference observed when a pH 1.5, 8.1, 11.9 solutions is measured against a pH5.5 solution as a reference. Inspection of these difference spectra are the due primarily to tyrosine and tryptophane. The spectrum which is ypical shown in these figures (2.18, 2.19, 2.20) give information regarding conformation from the following ways:

(a) the sign of the difference spectrum is positive. This usually signifies that a number of amino acids are exposed to the pH in the reference than in the sample, i, e., that the amino acids on HSA become more exposed as the pH decreased from 5.5. (b) the types of amino acuts involved and the number of them may be deterined the perturbation phenolic produces difference spectrum peaks at 280 and 288 nm and perturbation of the tryptophan chromophores produces difference spectrum peak at 295 nm.

Effect of some drugs on albumin absorption spectra:

Table (2.8) and fig (2.17) show that λmax of albumin bound with each of thyroxine, oleic acid and cortisol separately. The data show that there was long shift in λmax when HSA is bound with thyroxine (T4) and two peaks were obtained at λmax of (291.8 and 258.6nm) due to the interaction between T4 and HSA molecules, causing to bring some phenylalanyl residues to the surface of albumin that gives the λmax 258.6 nm.

Thyroxine molecule have a high electron density which cause a high effect on the tyrosyl absorbance peak. HAS has a high binding capacity for several other hormones such as those of the following at the respected percentage of cortisol 30% thyroxine 10% and long chain fatty acids such as locate, plamitate…etc to about 99.9% (190). These findings of formation of L-T4-HSA complex suggested a structural changes in HSA molecules have occurred whereas oleic acid bound to HSA caused no affect on the structure of the HSA but a high wave-length of λmax of tyrosine oleic acid was obtained. When cortisol was bound to HSA, refolding of HSA was resulted bringing all tyrosyl residues to the down surface (buried) of the molecules these results indicate that all chromophoric amino acid are buried interiorly, so there is no significant absorption peak happened on the spectra as shown in fig 2.15.

Spectrophotomric titration of HSA:

Many studies of protein structure require the determination of pK values for proton dissociation from ionizable amino acid side chain because these values give an indication of the location of the amino acid in protein according to the following rule, for example for, amino acids and always increase if atitratable group (e.g, the OH of tyrosine imndazole of histidine, and SH of eysteine) is charged. Hence, when the pH is changed:-

(a) if no spectral chanfe is observed for one of these cromophores and if the pH change is such the titration of free am bo acid would have occurred, the chromophore must be buried in anon polar region of the protein.

(b) if the spectral change as function of pH indicates that the ionizable group has the same pK as it would be free in solution, when amino acid is on the surface of the protein.

(c) if the spectral change as afunction of pH indicates avery different pK, then the amino acid is likely to be in strongly polar environment (e.g. atyrosine surrounded by carboxyl group). This can often be done spectrophotometerically because dissociation often changes the spectrum of one of chromophores (e.g. tyrosine) see fig (2.4). if we apply this rule to determine the noumber of external tyrosines and if all are on the surface and they are ionized by increasing the pH, the entur tyrosine spectrum will shift to that seem in fig (2.4) for free tyrosine at high pH value. In other words a plot of absorbance at λmax =295nm against pH values would look like the eurve in fig (2.21). from this eurve one can conclude that about 30% of the tyrosyl residues located on the surface of the protein (HSA) while the other 70% were buried interior the albumin folded structure at the native form.

These results have given a considerable attention on the role of tyrosl residues in the structure and reactions of HSA (204-209). In addition the results obtained in this chapter indicates that the albumin posses various advantage, e.g. their amino acid composition has a high ratio of tysyl to tryptopgyls.

Table (2.1): effect of pH on the λmax of the purified HSA (as explained in 2.2.3.1 in the text).

pH	λmax (nm)
1.6	276.6
7.0	278.0
8.0	280.0

9.0	282.8
10.0	286.4
12.0	295.3

Table (2.2): absorption maxima (λmax) for tyrosine and phenylalanine, the effect was carried out at different pH, (as explaned in 2.2.3.1 in the text).

Chromophor	pH	Λmax(nm)
Tyrosine	1.6	274.6233.2
=	7.0	274.8 233.4
=	12.6	293.0
Phenylalanine	1.6	257.6 216.6
=	7.0	258.0 216.6
=	12.6	258.2 221.4

Table (2.3) effect of 10% ethanol on the λmax of HSA , tyrosine and phenylalanine, all other details are outlined in the text

Sample	pH	Λmax (nm)
HSA	1.7	276.0
HSA	6.9	277.8
HSA	12.6	291.2 258.0
phy	1.7	249.4 219.6
phy	6.9	258.0 252.2
phy	12.6	258.6
Tyr	1.7	250.6 2.0

Tyr	6.9	250.6 225.8
Tyr	12.6	294.6 241.8

Table (2.4): the effect of ethylene glycol concentration on λmax of HSA at pH 7.0, all other details are explaine in the text.

% ethylene glycole	Λmax (nm)
5	278
10	283
20	287
25	288
30	291

Table (2.5): the effect of polarity on the λmax of HSA at nutral pH region, (as explained in section 2.2.3.2 in the text.)

Solvent	λmax(nm)
20% PEG	278.4
50% PEG	278.2
20% glycerol	278.4
50% glycerol	278.4
20% DMSO	300.0, 276.2
20% dioxane	277.8, 232.8
50% dioxane	277.6, 236.4

Table (2.6): the effect of urea and KCI on the λmax of HSA spectra at different pH values (as explained in section 2.2.3.2)

Solvent	pH	Λmax(nm)
8.M urea	7.0	278.6
8M urea	3.8	299.6, 263.0
8M urea+0.03M.KCI	6.2	299.4, 295.6
0.03M KCI	7.0	300.0, 261.6

Table (2.7) difference spectra of albumin vs tyrosine and phenvalanine mixture at neutral, acidic and basic media. All other dentratre explained in section 2.2.3

pH	Λmax(nm)
1.6	286.6, 236.6
7.0	287.4, 236.4
12.6	259.0, 224.0

Table (2.8) effect of some drugs on the HSA. All other detaik are explained in section 2.2.3.3, in the text.

Sample	λmax(nm)
HSA –thyroxine	291.8, 258.6
HSA cortesol	- -
HSA oleic acid	298.8

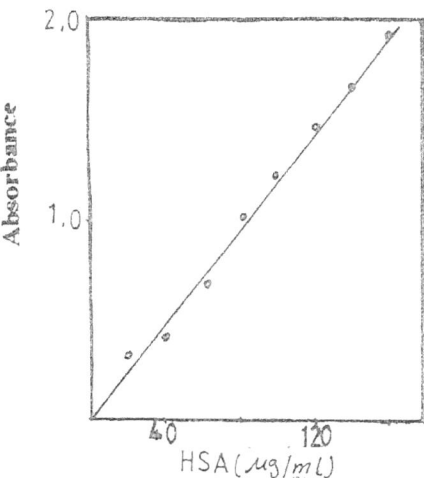

Fig (2.1) standard curve of protein determination by lowry methed (usin HSA as standard).

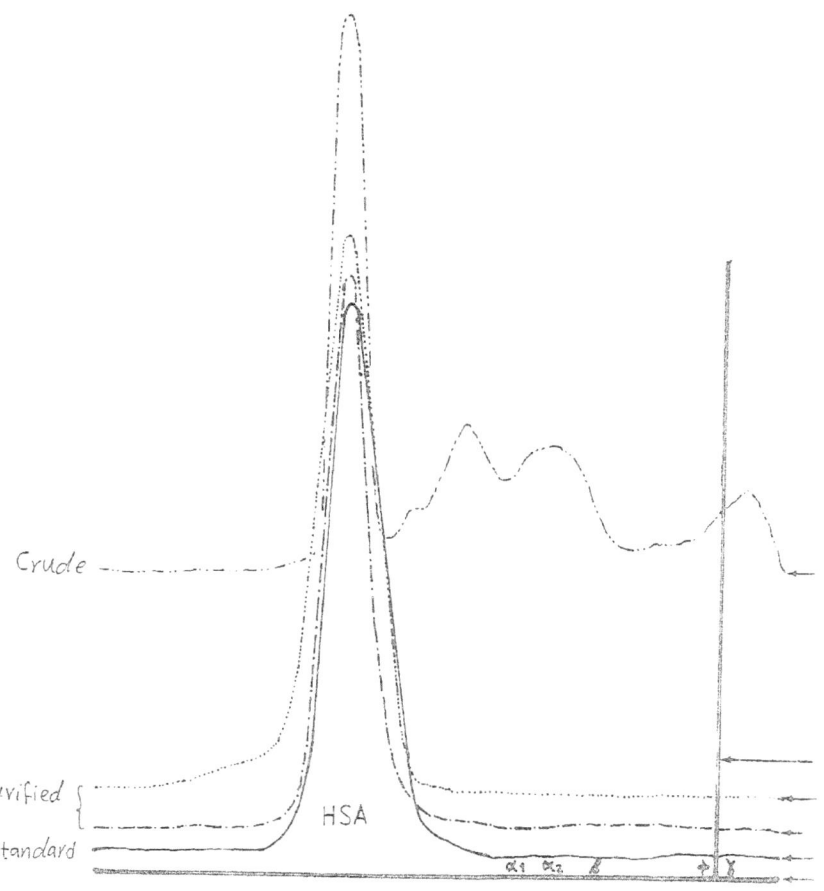

Fig (2.2) electrophoresis profile for crude serum purified HSA standard HSA all are explained in the text.

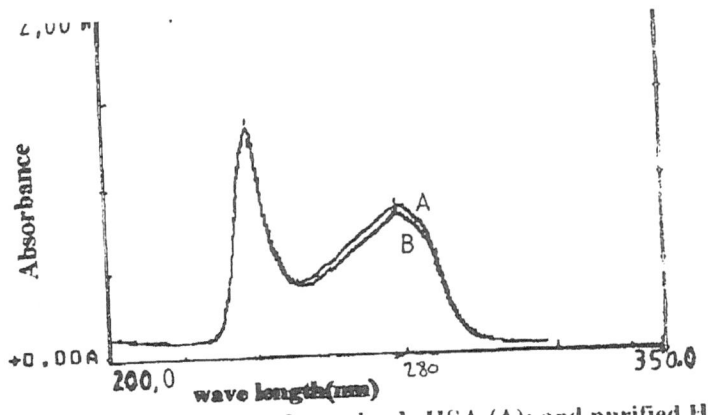

Fig (2.3) Absorption spectra of standard HSA (A); and purified HSA(B .All details are outlined in the text.

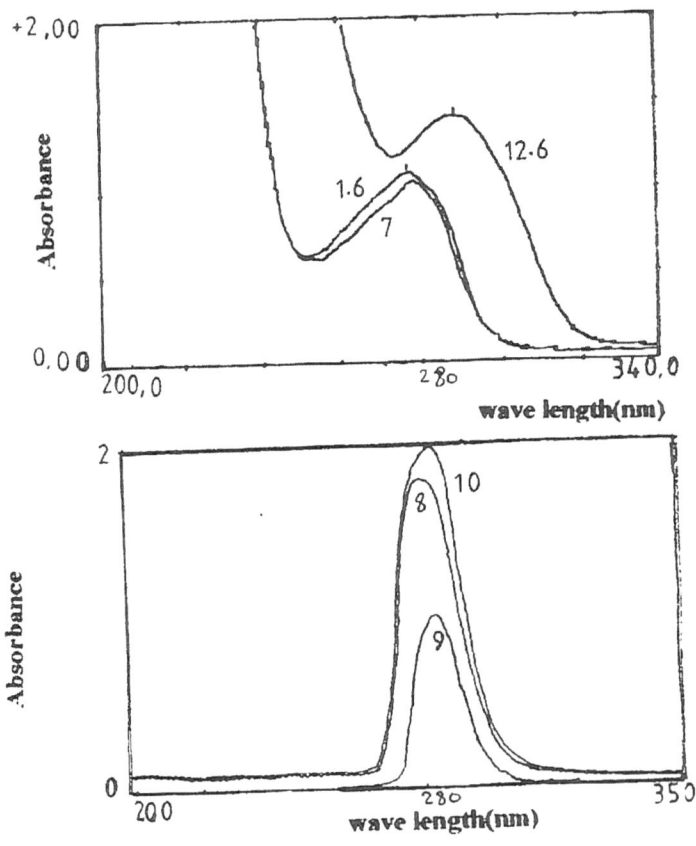

Fig (2.4) pH dependence of difference spectral results for purified HSA using phosphate buffer all detail are explained in the text,

80

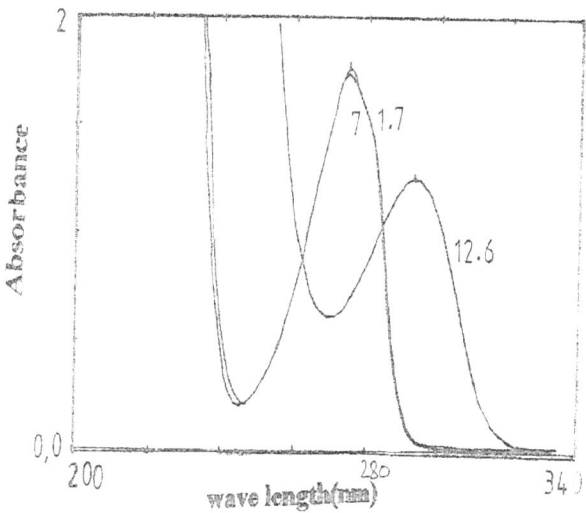

Fig (2.5) pH dependence of tyrosine spectrum using phosphate buffer. All details are explained in the text.

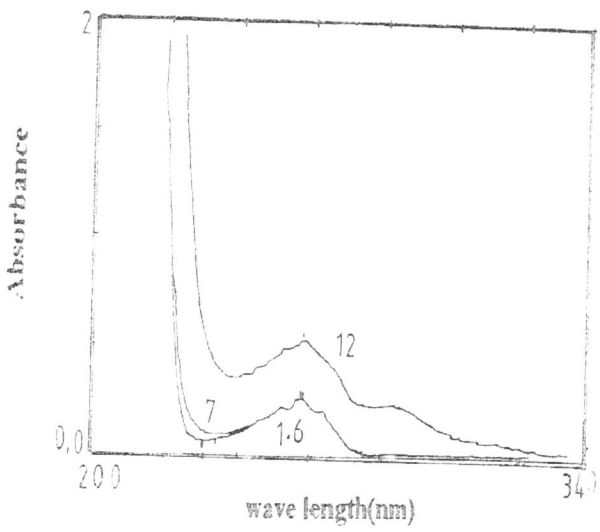

Fig (2.6) pH dependence of phenylalanine spectra using phosphate buffer. All details are explained in the text

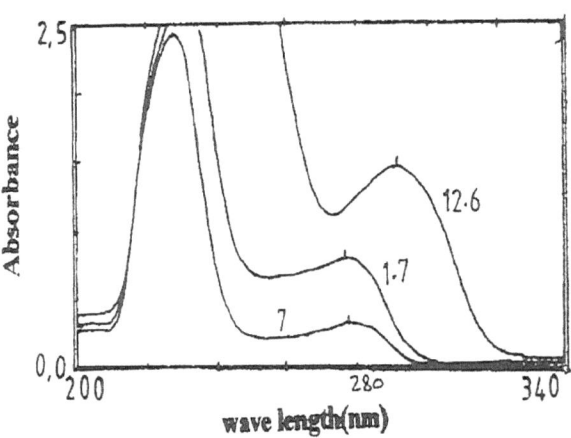

Fig (2.7) Absorbance spectrum of albumin in 10% ethanol: water mixture at different pH. regions .All details are explained in the text.

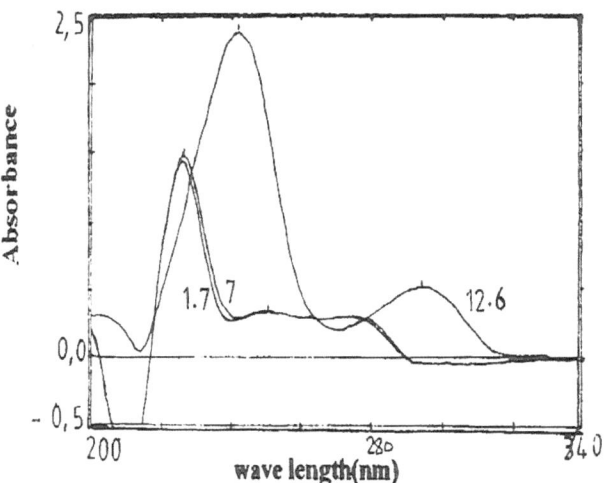

Fig (2.8, a) the effect of 10% ethanol on, tyrosine spectrum at different pH values (1.7, 7.0 and 12.6). all derails are explained in the text.

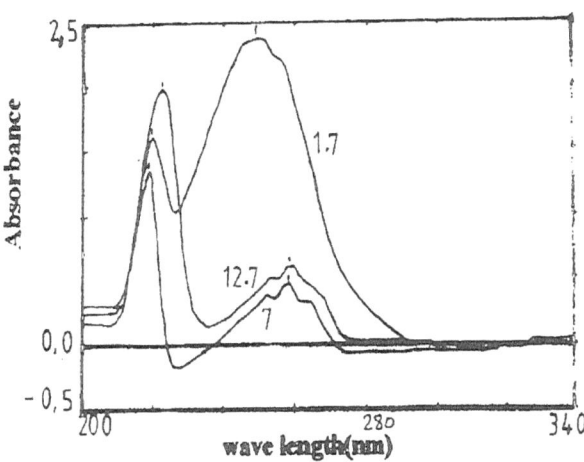

Fig (2.8,b) The effect of 10% ethanol on: phenylalanine. absorbance at pH (1.7 , 7,and 12.6).All details are outlined in the text.

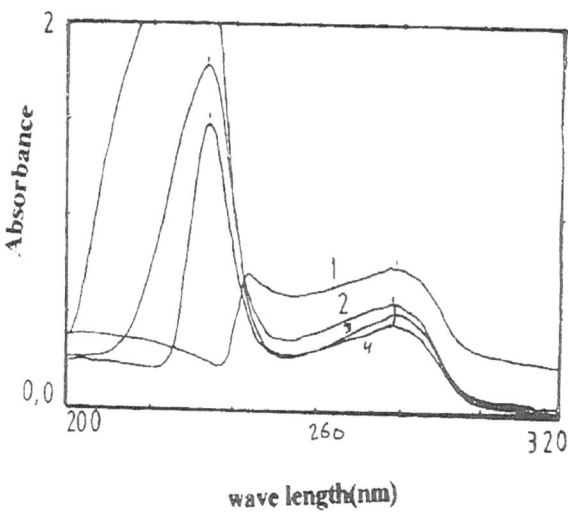

Fig (2.9) albumin spectra in 20% of (1) glycerol, (2) dioxane, (3) DMSO and (4) polyethylene glycol at (pH 7.0). all details explained in the text.

83

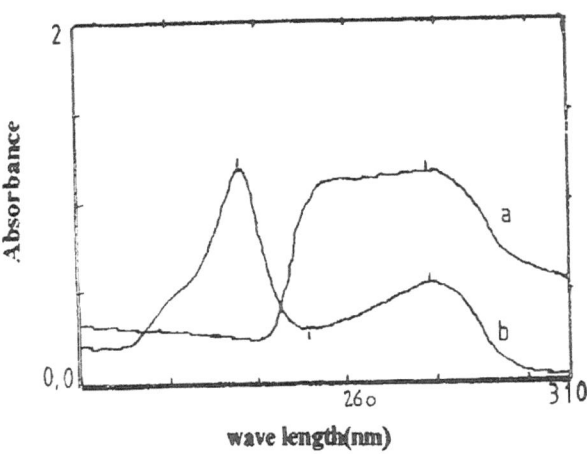

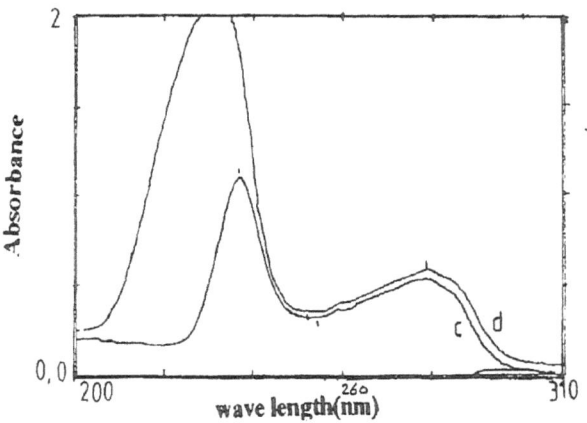

Fig (2.10) the effect of 50% DMSO (a) and 50% PEG (b), dioxane (c) and glycerol (d) on the albumin spectra at neutral Ph. All details are explained in the text,

84

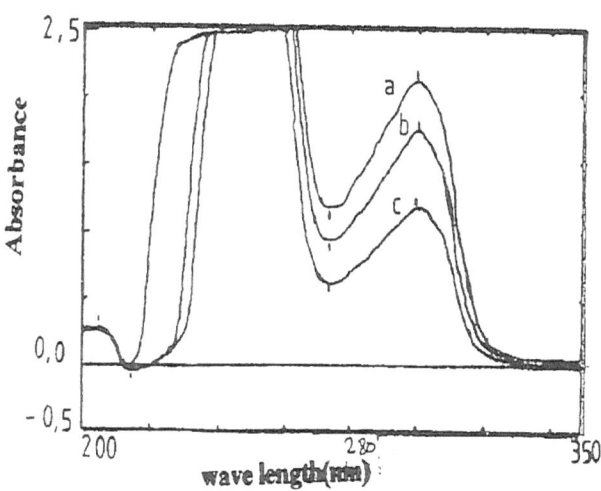

Fig (2.11) Spectera of albumin in (a) 8molar urea ,(b)0.O3M KCl,(c)8M
urea +0.O3M Kcl solution . All details are explained in the text .

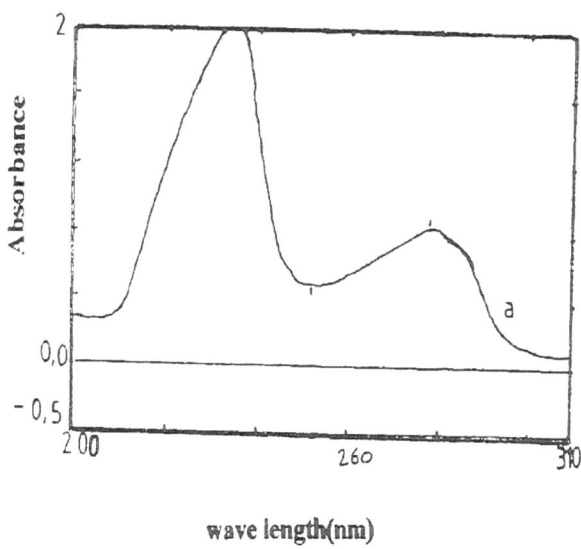

Fig (2.12) The effect of urea concentration on the albumin absorbance at
pH 7.0 (a) 20% urea (b) 50% urea . All details are outlined in the
text.

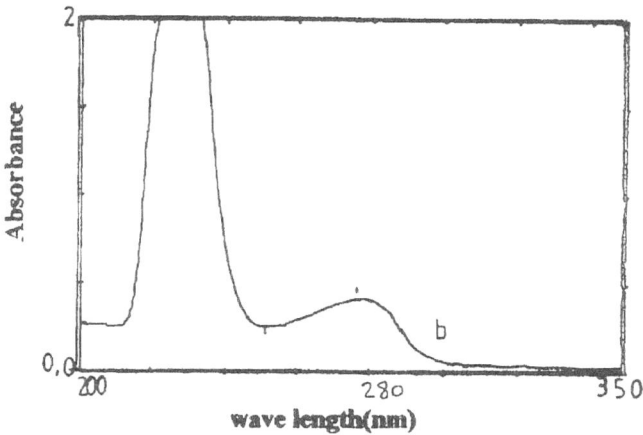

Fig (2 12 b)

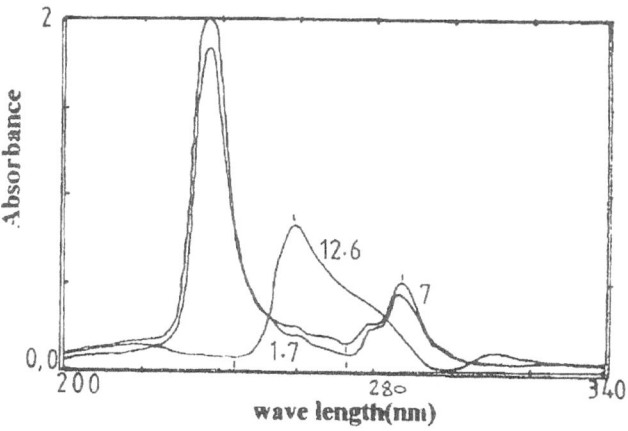

Fig (2.13) the difference spectra obtained with HSA solution in the sample beam and tyrosine + phenylalanine mixture in the reference beam. At different pH values. All details are explained in the text.

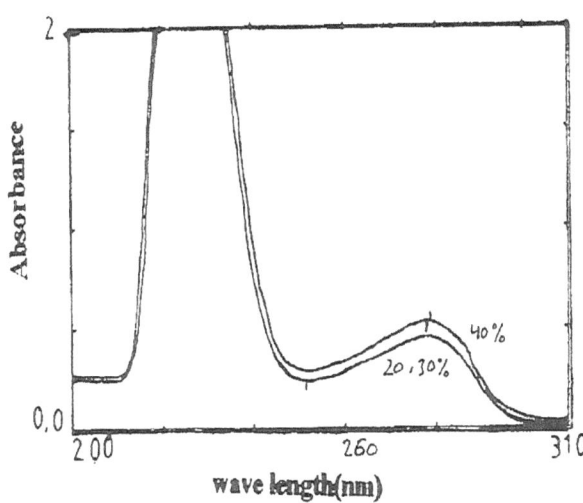

Fig (2.14) The effect of urea concentration on HSA absorbance spectrum ,HSA in H₂O (in Ref.beam) HSA in urea (20,30,40)% (in sample beam). All details are explained in the text.

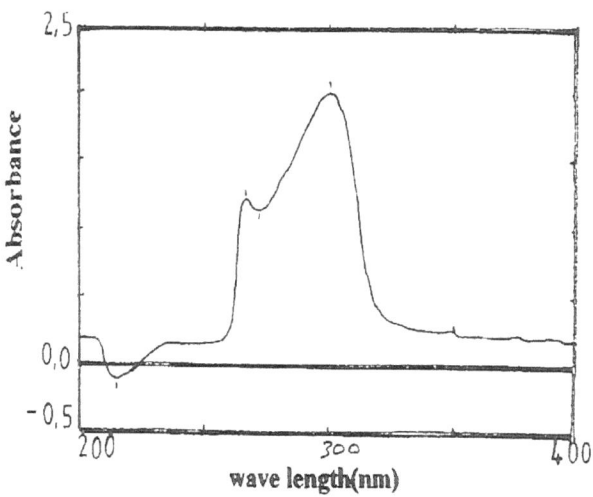

Fig (2.15) the effect of polarity on the HAS spectra. HAS in H2O (pH.7.0) (in ref. beam). HAS in 20% DMSO (in sample beam). all details are outlined in the text.

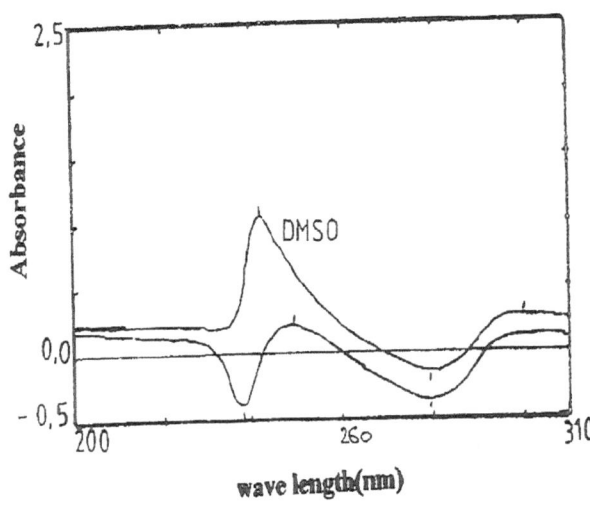

Fig(2.16.A) The effect of PEG and DMSO on the HSA absorbance
HSA in: PEG and DMSO . All details are explained in the text

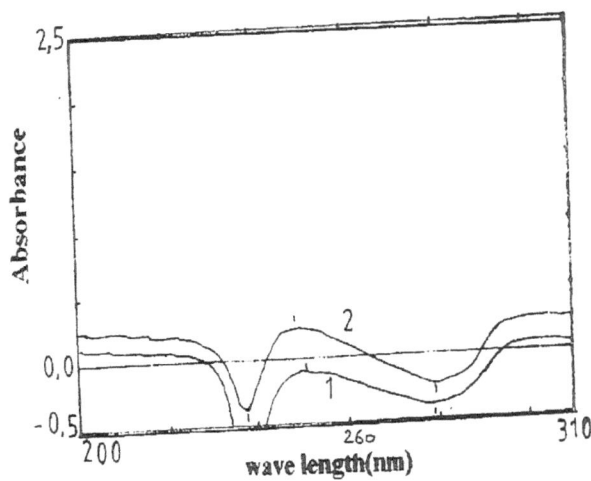

Fig (2.16, b) the effect of glycerol and dioxane (20%) on the albumin spectra, HSA IN H2O in reference cell. HAS in (20% glycerol (1) 20% dioxane (2) in sample cell).

88

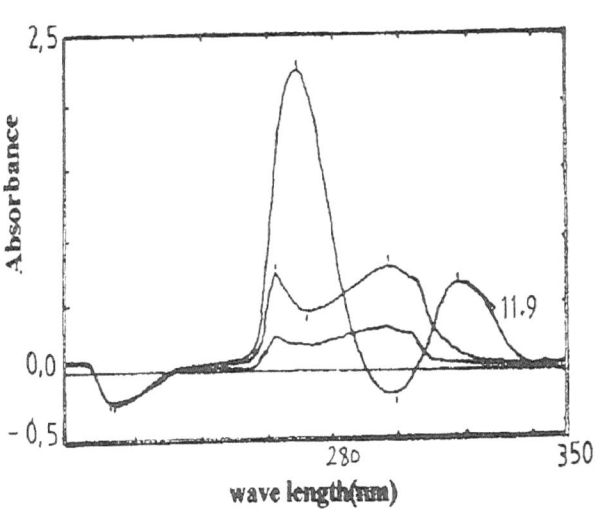

Fig(2.19) As explained in Fig (2.18) but, HSA, pH 6.8 ref. cell, HSA pH
1.5 and 11.9 in Sample cell. All details are explained in the text.

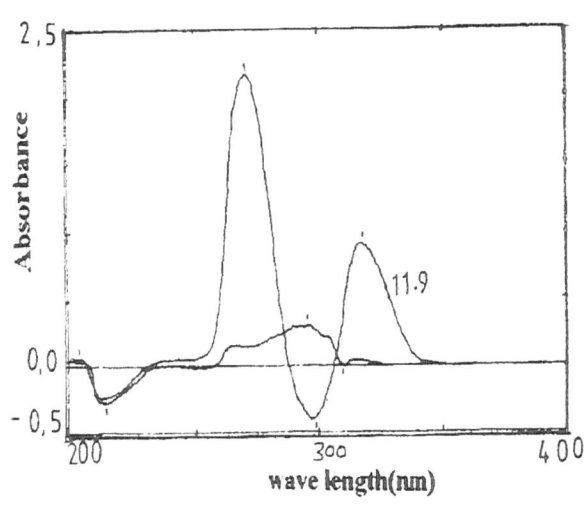

Fig.(2.20) As explained in Fig (2.19) but, HSA pH 7.0 in ref. cell, HSA pH
1.5, 11.9 in sample cell. All details are explained in the text.

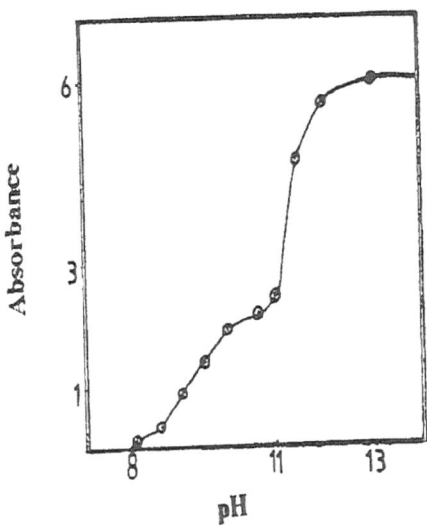

Fig(2.21) The titration curve of purified albumin at different pH.
(λ_{max} 295 nm).

Development of a method for binding of ^{99}Tc-MDP to the human albumin (HSA).

SUMMARY

This chapter deals with the binding of 99mTc-MDP to the purified human serum albumin (HSA). the specificity of 99mTc-MDP binding to 21-23% of the total binding. The range of optimum pH for the binding was 7.4-7.6. the most suitable amounts for HSA to give maximum binding was (70μg) per incubation medium, binding seemed to be affected by 99mTc-MDP concentration and also mono and divalent chloride salts. The association constants (ka) and maximum binding capacity (Bmax) of ^{99m}Tc-MDP binding to binding sites of HSA was determined from scatchard and double reciprocal plots, the results revealed that Ka and Bmax values were temperature dependent.

INTERODUCTION

Normaly nearly many drugs, fatty acids and hormones...etc are transport through the human body by serum albumin, plasma lobg-chain fatty acid, such as oleate, plamitate, linoleate, stearate and phospholipid are transported in association with serum albumin (229). Albumin binds 1-2 fatty acid molecules to form a stable complex, this association stabilizes the fat and confers increased stability on the protein. About 99.9% bilirubin and long chain fatty acid are though to be albumin bound in normal plasma, this is important in neonates in whom entry into the brain tissue is cause of bilirubin encephalopathy in neonatal jaundice and depends on the level of free plasma bilirubin (230.

Many hormones are bound to plasma albumin and indicate percentage bound in normal plasma:-

Cortesol 30%, corticosterone (30%), thyroxine (10%), aldosterone (60%), testo sterone (60%), other substances known to bind with albumin are bile pigments, prostaglandins, some amino acid, triiodo thyronine, urate, salicylate, penicillin, ampicillin and other antibioties, drugs including barbiturate, sulphonamides, disphenyl hydantion, worfarin...etc. (231). Theoretical and paractical aspects of the interaction of therapeutic drugs with transport proteins in human blood have been considered, during the last decade more attention was paid to diagnostic radiolabelled compounds especially the technetium complexes which have become the most frequently used radiopharmaceuticals (232). Understanding the mechanism of their biolocalization in specific target organ tissues, as well as. Their elimination (generally-theirbiokneties) may depend on elucidation of their biochemical characteristics such as protein binding and specific protein binding (binding to individual circulatory proteins). In this chapter method was developed to study the binding of HSA to ^{99m}Tc-MDP.

3.1 INSTRUMENTS AND CHEMICALS USED

3.1.1 instruments used:

1- LKB gama counter type 1270-rack gama II was used to measure the radioactivity emitted by 99mTc isotope.

2- hetashi (U-2000) spectrophotometer.

3-pye-unicam pH meter.

4-memmert water bath.

5-pye-unicam digital pH meter.

3.1.2 materials used:

3.1.2.1 general chemicals:

All laboratory chemical and reagents used in thes work were of analar grad unless otherwise specified and were obtained from fluka company, Switzerland ($CaCl2$, $Na_2HPO_4.XH_2O$, $MgCl_2$, NaH_2PO_4), KCI, NaOH, NaCI, $SnCI_2.2H_2O$ from BDH, Limited, pool U.K, methylene diphosphonate (MDP) from ORDH company, germany, sephadex, G100 from pharmacia fine chemicals, Switzerland.

3.1.2.2 phosphate buffer:

Phosphate buffer was prepared by dissolving the appropriate amount of salts (Na_2HPO, $7H_2O$ OR $Na_2HPO4.12H_2O$ and NaH_2PO_4) in distilled water and the required pH was adjusted.

Stock solutions:

0.2 m dibasic sodium phosphate (53.65g $NaHPO_4.7H_2O$ or 71.7g of $Na_2HPO_4.12H_2O$ in 1000ml) , 0.2 m monobasic sodium phosphate (27.8g NaH_2PO_4 in 1000ml). the required pH was prepared by mixing an accurate volumes of stock solution, then the pH was checked by pye-unicam digital pH-meter.

3.2 PRELIMINARY TEST FOR THE BINDING OF 99MTC-MDP TO THE HSA

3.2.1 preparation of ^{99m}Tc-MDP

a- methylene diphosphon (MDP) kit:

the MDP kit was prepared according to the following (233):

1- 1.25g MDP was dissolved in 200ml nitrogen-parged distilled water in closed flask and stored under nitrogen pressure.

2- 0.6g $SnCl_2.2H_2O$ dissolved in slightly acidified distilled water with 0.1N-HCI, then after dissolving the solution was transferred to closed cial and stored under N_2-gas pressure to prevent the oxidation of $SnCI_2$ to $SnCI_4$.

3- 2.5ml of $SnCI_2$ solution was added dropewise with continuous stirring to the MDP solution, the solution should be clear, the pH of the solution must be adjusted to 6 using 1N-NaOH.

4- The final solution was filtered through Millipore filter and 1ml aliquots of the filtered solution was placed in vial under N_2-gas pressure and then lyophilized.

b-technetium generator (300mci) was purchased from amersham bucks, England supplied by Iraqi atomic energy commissiom (IAEC).

3.2.2 sephadex-G100 preparation:

1- the gel was prepared by swelling 10mg of sephadex G-100 IN 100ml of 50m M phosphate buffer pH 7.4 for 24 hours at room temperature (about 30°c) then stored a4 4°c to equilibrate it with the buffer.

2- the suspension was carefully mixed before pouring into vertical column (with diameter of 1.0cm) contaning eluant buffer. After the gel has sttled, the column outlet was opened. Packing was continued until the gel reached stable bed height (30cm) then the column was equilibrated with 50m M phosphate buffer pH7.4 with flow rate of 12ml per hour, then sample (500μl) was applied to the surface of the gel carefully to sparate bound ^{99m}Tc-MDP (^{99m}Tc-MDP-HSA complex) from the free. Elution was carried out using the same buffer of equilibration with flow eate of 12ml per hour and fraction volume of 2ml.

3.3 LABELLING OF HSA WITH 99MTC

1- MDP kit contain (5mg MDP and 0.5mg $SnCl_2$) was dissolved in 5ml phosphate buffer and left for 15 minutes before labelling MDP concentration was 2.8×10^{-3}M, the other concentrations were prepared by serial dilution from this concentration using phosphate buffer pH 7.4.

2- 10μci ^{99m}Tc eluted with saline from the ^{99m}Tc-generator, was added to the MDP solution, incubated for 15 minutes then 100μl of HSA solution (750μg/ml) was added and incubated to the required time (15, 20, 30, 45 & 60) or required temperature (20, 30, 37, 50 and 60°c).

3- the sample was then applied to the surface of sephadex G-100 gel filteration column which prepared in 3.2.2, elution was carried out using the same buffer to separate bound 99mTc-MDP-HSA complex from free ^{99m}Tc-MDP with flow rate of 12ml/h and fraction volume of 2ml. accordingly three types of sample were applied to the surface of the same column by the following procedures.

(a) ^{99m}Tc:

10μl of ^{99m}Tc was diluted to 500μl with phosphate buffer pH 7.4, then was added to the surface of the same column used in the sparation of ^{99m}Tc-MDP-HSA complex, elution was carred out using the same buffer, the radioactive of each fraction was measured by gamma counter expressed in counts per minute (cpm).

Calculation:

The radioactivity of each fraction was plotted vs corresponding fraction number.

c- ^{99m}Tc-MDP-HSA :

1-10μl ^{99m}Tc was added to 100μl MDP (2.8×10^{-6}M), incubated for 15 minutes at 25c.

2-100μl of HSA (1mg/ml) was then added to ^{99m}Tc-MDP solution the finl volume was completed to 500μl with phosphate buffer inclubated for 30minat 25c.

3-the solution was then added on the surface of the same column. And then eluted with same buffer.

4-the fraction volume 2ml were collected with flow rate of 12ml/h.

5-the activity of each fraction was neasured with gamma counter.

6-the spectrum at wave length (200-300nm) of the same fractions collected in step (4) were measured.

Calculation :

1- the radioactivity of each fraction was plotted vs corresponding fraction number.

2- the absorbance of each fraction was plotted vs its crrespunding fraction number.

3.4 MOST APPROPARATE CONDITIONS OF ^{99}MTC BINDING TO HSA

3.4.1 choice of the most appropriate amount of the HSA for the pinding of ^{99m}Tc-MDP:

1- 100µl containing different amount of HSA (0.3, 0.5, 0.8, 1.00, 1.1 and 1.3mg/ml stock solution) were pipetted into RIA tubes 100µl ^{99m}Tc-MDP solution then was added o each tubes of HSA solution, the reaction mixture was incubated for 30 minutes at 25c the final volume was completed to 500µl using phosphate buffer pH 7.4.

2- the samples were applied to the surface of the sephadex G-100 gl filteration column (1x30cm) equilibrated with phosphate buffer pH 7.4 elution was carred out using the same above buffer, the separate bound ^{99m}Tc-MDP-HSA complex from free ^{99m}Tc-MDP, with flow rate of 12ml/h and fraction volumes of (2ml).

3- radioactivity of each fraction tube in cpm was counted using gamma counter.

4- the steps from 1-3 were repeated with the addition of 100µl of unlabelled gloucoheptonate (GH) with concentrations ranging from $1.4x10^4$ to $2.8x10^{-4}$M (50-100 times ore than MDP).

Calculation :

1- total binding (TB) represents the amount of radioactivity bound to the particulate fraction (cpm) in the absence of unlablled GH.

2- The radioactivity of the particulate fraction after the maximum displacement of the labelled MDP by excess Amount of unlabelled GH is referred to as nonspecific binding (NB).

3- specific binding (SB) is the difference between radioactivity (cpm) bound to the particulate fraction in the absence of excess unlabelled GH (IB) and that bound in its presence (NB).

SB (CPM) = TB (CPM)-NB (CPM)

$$SB\% = \frac{SB(CPM)}{\text{total count}(CPM) \text{ of labelled MDP used in each tube}(TC)} \times 100$$

5- The value of SB% corresponding to amount of albumin used was plotted vs HSA concentration (mg).

3.4.2 effect of pH on the binding of the 99mTc-MDP to HSA:

1- 100µl albumin (1mg/ml) was incubated with 100µl 99mTc-MDP (2.8×10^{-6}M) at 25c for 30 minutes. The final volume was 500µl using phosphate buffer a different pH ranging from 7.0 to 8.0.

2- the steps 2-4 of experiment 3.4.1 were followed.

Calculation:

1- the same mathematical formula mentioned in experiment 3.4.1 was used to calculate specific binding SB%.

2- specific Binding (SB%) was converted to bound ^{99m}Tc-TDP in molarity according to the follwing formula:

Specifically bound = SB% X total ^{99m}Tc-MDP concentration
^{99m}Tc-MDP in (molar)   in incubation media (M)

3- Specifically bound ^{99m}Tc-MDP in molar was plotted vs their corresponding Ph.

3.4.3 choice of the most appropriate amount of MDP for the binding of 99mTc-MDP with HSA:

1- 100μl of HSA (1mg/ml) was added to 100μl of each MDP concentration ranging from 2.8×10^{-3} to 2.8×10^{-9} molar, the total volume was completed to 500μl with phosphate buffer pH 7.4, and incubated for 30 minutes at room temperature (abou 30c).

2- the steps 2-4 of experiment 3.3 were followed.

Calculation :

1-specific binding (SB%) of each MDP concentration was determined as in experiment 3.4.1.

2- the percent of specifically bound ^{99m}Tc-MDP of each concentration was plotted against MDP concentration in incubation media.

3.4.4 effect of monovalent and divalent salts on binding of ^{99m}Tc-MDP to HSA :

3.4.4.1 Effect of monovalent salts:

1- 100µl of albumin solution (1mg/ml) was incubated with 100µl of ^{99m}Tc-MDP (2.8×10^{-6}M) at about 30c for 30 minutes, in presence of different concentration of NaCI or KCI (50-250mM) and final volume 500µl completed with pH 7.4.

2- steps 2-4 of experiment 3.4.1 were repeated.

Calculation :

1- specific binding % at each salt concentration was determined as in experiment 3.4.1.

2- the amount of specifically bund ^{99m}Tc-MDP at each salt concentration was determined as experiment 3.4.2.

3- the amount of specifically bound ^{99m}Tc-MDP (in molar) were plotted against the ionic strength or concentration of the salts in the incubation media.

3.4.4.2 effect of divalent chloride salts:

1- 100µl of albumin (1mg/ml) solution was incubated with 100µl ^{99m}Tc-MDP solution (2.8×10^{-6}M) at about 30c for 30 minutes at pH 7.4 in presence of different concentrations (50-250mm) of $CaCI_2$ and $MgCI_2$ final volume was 500µl.

2- steps 2-4 of experiment 3.4.1 were repeated.

Calculation :

1- specific binding % of each salt concentration was calculated as in experiment 3.4.1.

2- the amount of specific binding in molar was calculated as in experiment 3.4.2

3- the values of specifically bound in molar were plotted vs salt concentration.

Solution:

(1) 1M-NaCI stock solution : 5.85g of NaCI was dissolved in 100ml hosphate buffer pH 7.4

(2) 1M-KCI stock solution : 7.45g of KCI was dissolved in 100ml phosphate buffer pH 7.4

(3) 1M-CaCI$_2$ stock solution : 11.0g of CaCI$_2$ was dissolved and made up to 100ml phosphate buffer pH 7.4

(4) 1M-MgCI$_2$ stock solution : 9.43 g MgCI$_2$ was dissolved and made up to 100ml by phosphate buffer pH 7.4

From this stock solution all other different cocentrations were prepared by serial dilution.

3.5 SATURATION EXPERIMENTS AND SCATCHARD ANALYSIS

1- 100μl HSA solution (1mg/ml) was incubated with increasing amount of ^{99m}Tc-MDP $(1.0-10.0) \times 10^{-7}$M, 100μl of each concentration was used, the final volume was completed to 500μl with phosphate buffer at pH 7.4

2- A paralled set of assay tubes were used to determine nonspecific binding as outlined in the previous experiments. The experiment was carried out in duplicate.

3- all of above tubes were incubated at 37°c and pH 7.4 for 30 minutes.

4- the steps 2 and 3 of experiment 3.4.1 were performed as outlined.

5- all the previous steps of the experiment were performed at different tempratures (20, 30 and 50°c).

Calculation :

1- B is the bound radioactivity (cpm) which represents the 99mTc-MDP-HSA complex. F is the free radioactivity (cpm) which represents non bound ^{99m}Tc-MDP.

F= total count (TC) – Bound radioactivity

2-the value of ^{99m}Tc-MDP which is bound specifically in molar were calculated using the following formua:-

$$B_{specific} = \frac{TB - NB}{TC} \times \text{concentration of } ^{99m}Tc - MDP(M) \text{ used in incubation media}$$

3- B$_{secific}$ was plotted vs concentration of ^{99m}Tc-MDP (M) used.

4- the plot of B/F values vs the values of B$_{secific}$ give alinear relationships. The value of the affinity constant of the binding at each remperature can be calculated from the slope of the straight line while the value of the total binding site concentration (B_{max}) was calculated from the relation:- $B/F = (1/K_d) (Bmax - B_{secific})$

5- K_d and Bmax values were also obtained from the double reciprocal plot of data getting from scachard lots, using the following formula (234).

$$\frac{1}{B_{specific}} = \left\{ \frac{K_d}{B_{max}} \times \frac{1}{[F]} \right\} + \frac{1}{B_{max}}$$

1/ $B_{secific}$ value were plotted vs 1/(f) x -1/K_d value was obtained from intercept on abscissa. 1/ B_{max} value was obtained from intercept on ordinate. Where (f) represent the free ^{99m}T-MDP in molar.

3.6 TEST OF OTHER BINDING PROTEINS WITH 99MTC-MDP

1- 100µl of each of , α , β, γ – gloubulin (750µg/ml) was incubated with 100µl ^{99m}Tc-MDP (2.8×1^{-6}M) in serial experiments, at 37°c for 30 minutes, te final volume was completed to 500µl with phosphate buffer pH 7.4

2- steps 2 and 3 of experiment 3.4.1 were repeated.

3- the radioactivity of each fraction (cpm) was measured, using gamma-counter.

Calculation:

The radioactivity (cpm) of each fraction was ploted vs corresponding number.

RESULTS AND DISCUSSION

Preliminary test for the binding of ^{99m}Tc-MDP to the HSA:

The purified albumin was used to study or investigate how the ^{99m}Tc-MDP binding was carried out. After 30 minutes of incubation at 30c, the bound ^{99m}Tc-MDP-HSA complex was sparated by gel filteration chromatography (235) using sephadex G-100 column (1x30cm). the bound 99mTc-MDP complex was observed in fractions 4-9, where the non bound was observed in the fractions 11-16. as shown in fig (3.1)

Fig (3.2) shows U.V spectra for four type of compounds MDP, ^{99m}Tc-MDP-HSA, 99mTc-MDP and HSA, ^{99m}Tc-MDP and MDP have the same spectra but differs from those of 99mTc-MDP-HSA and HSA , the last two compounds differ in the λmax (278.8, 253.5, 219.4 nm for 99mTc-MDP-HSA and 278.1, 253.1, 215.1nm for HSA). the results indicate that the bound ^{99m}mTc-MDP-HSA is new compound results from binding of ^{99m}mTc-MDP- to HSA.

These results have helped in the identification of fractions eluted from the column chromatography fig (3.1), the eluted bound ^{99m}Tc-MDP-HAS complex was observed in the earlier fractions (4-9) wherease non bound ^{99m}Tc-MDP appear in the fractions eluted later, the specificity of the binding was investigated by introducing different concentrations of unlabeled glucoheptonate (GH) into incubation medium. The concentration of the unlabelled GH (M) which was necessary to cause a maximum displacement of the ^{99m}Tc-MDP equals 100 times that of ^{99m}Tc-MDP concentration (M). about 77.79% of the bound ^{99m}Tc-MDP was displaced from its binding proteins (HSA), hence the nonspecific binding for HSA was 21.23%. the amount of nonspecificity remained constant what ever higher concentrations of the unlabelled GH used, as in fig (3.3). Ortega and mas-oliva determined the non-specific binding of ^{125}I-CaM to cardiac sarcolema using unlabelled CaM with concentration higher than that of ^{125}I-CaM by 166 times (236), while olsen et al. used unlablled aM with concentration of 2500 times more than ^{125}I-CaM concn. For maximum displacement of ^{125}I-CaM bound to secretory granules of bovine neurohypophyses and the nonspecificity ranged between 9-14% of total bound (237). Sobue etal used 5mm EGTA for determination of non-specific binding and 5mm Ca$_{+2}$ for total binding, the former was less than 2% of the total binding (238).

The most appropriate conditions of ^{99m}Tc-MDP binding to its binding HSA :

The study of the binding of any ligand to its receptor or carrier necessitates the choice of the most appropriate conditions that lead to the maximum specific binding, hence the study of appropriate amount of HSA, the pH., MDP concentration, salt concentrations, time and temperature on the extent of the binding of ^{99m}Tc-MDP to its binding site in HSA is quite necessary.

The most appropriate amount of the HSA for the binding of ^{99m}Tc-MDP:

The specific binding of ^{99m}Tc-MDP to HSA was enhanced with increasing amount of HSA, fig (3.4). 100μg-110μg HSA gave the maximum value of the specific binding, this means that the depletion in the HSA concentration in the blood such as in the case of albuminanimia (239) effect the binding of ^{99m}Tc-MDP and lead to give various pattern of bone scanninh depending on the concentration of HSA.

Effect of pH on the binding of ^{99m}Tc-MDP to its binding HSA:

Fig (3.5) show the effect of increasing pH from 7.0 to 8.0 on the binding of ^{99m}Tc-MDP to is binding sites of HSA, maximum value of the specific binding occurred at 7.4-7.6 (exhibits a narrow pH-optimum), the results indicated that the binding was pH-dependent and the shift in the pH of environment may affect the properties of the HSA involved in binding. This effect includes the inducation of protonation-deprotonation process occurring within the ionizabic groups of the amino acids present in the binding domain of these macro molecules (240), so protonation-eproton reaction are important in ^{99m}Tc-MDP interaction with its binding HSA and the ionic or electrostatic interactions may take part in stabilization of the complex (241). Our results are similar in case of optimum pH to that obtained by huigen Y.M. etal. (167).

Effect of MDP concentration on the binding HSA :

Fig (3.6) show the effect of increasing amount of MDP on the binding of 99mTc-MDP to HSA, the total binding was increased to reach maximum bound at MDP concentration at 2.8×10^{-6} M-MDP and 2.2×10^{-7} M-SnCI2 as reducing agent, the increasing of MDP and SnCI2 concentrations may leads to a decrease in the total binding, these may be due to the dissociation of ^{99m}Tc-MDP complex. Our results are nearly similar to that obtained by Grouls etal (157).

Effect of monovalent and divalent salts on the binding of ^{99m}Tc-MDP to HSA :

When monovalent salts (NaCI and KCI) and divalent salts (CaCI₂ and MgCI₂) were added with different concentration (50-250mm) to the reaction mixture the results obtained indicated no significant effect on the ^{99m}Tc-MDP binding with HSA, as in fig (3.7 (A and B) show small decrease in the specific binding results from the effect of NaCI and KCI salts on the binding of ^{99m}Tc-MDP with HSA. fig (3.7 (C and D) show the effect of divalent salts (MgCI₂ and CaCI₂) on the specific binding, these results may be due to the interaction between [99mTc]-MDP and the cations of the salt, then equilibrium was reached near 120mm. the curves of fig (3.7) (A, B, C and D) indicate that a small amount of salt cause a high specific binding of [99mTc]-MDP to HSA , any further increasing in salt concentration more than 50mm cause instability of the [99mTc]-MDP-HSA complex, the reason may be due to the electrostatic interactions. Indeed if hydrophobic interactions were the force which stabilizing. [99mTc]-MDP-HSA , then increasing ionic strength would be expected to facilitate [99mTc]-MDP-HSA interactions.

In general, the mechanism by which these salts dissociate protein-protein complex is not completely clear, one hypothesis assumes that salts may alter the nature of the hydrophobic forces controlling the stabilization of protein –proten complex formed (242). The high concentrations of the salts tend to destabilize the complexes as a result of their interaction with water molecules leading to diminution of protein-protein interaction and reversible denaturtion of the protein (243, 244).

Saturation experiments and scatchard analysis:

The total binding of [99mTc]-MDP to HSA was increased as MDP concentration was increased reaching equilibrium, where the amount of bound 99mTc-MDP become nearly constant and the saturation of the binding sites on the HSA with [99mTc]-MDP molecules was achived as shown in fig (3-9), addition of [99mTc]-

MDP in the range (1×10^{-7} to 1.0×10^{-6}m) give a linear binding relation ship, the additional amount of MDP more than 5.8×10^{-6}m cause decreases in the binding with HSA, this may be due to the dissociation of ^{99m}Tc-MDP which affect the HSA binding or may be due to form adimer of ^{99m}Tc-MDP molecules (245). Table (3.1) show the amount of specifically bound ^{99m}Tc-MDP at equilibrium at 20, 30, 37 and 50c. these results indicate that the mount of bound ^{99m}Tc-MDP is temperature dependent and increases from 2.9×10^{-8} to 7.4×10^{-8} M with changing the temperature from (20 to 50) c, indicating that the reaction is slightly endothermic. Scatchard analysis (246) was used to determine the dissociation constant (K_d) and maximum binding capacities (Bmax) of ^{99m}Tc-MDP to human albumin by the following equation:

$B/F = (1/K_d) (B_{max} - B_{specific})$

As shown in fig (3-10), the value of B_{max} and Kd for HSA binding at different temperature are shown in table (3.2), B_{max} is a temperature dependant, increasing temperature from 20c to 50c, B_{max} increase about 1.8 fold, this can be explained according to that the number of molecules possessing the activation energy for interaction, increase with temperature. The Ka value are also temperature dependant, rising the temperature from (20 to 50) c the Ka values increase (1.13 times) this indicates that the reactions is slightly endothermic eactions enhanced by increasing temperature.

The Kd values were also temperature dependant, K_d and B_{max} values also deterined from double reciprocal plot according to fig (3.11), the results have compared with that obtained from scatchard plot (table 3.3) and showed similar values. From these results we an conclude that the Kd and B_{max} values of ^{99m}Tc-MDP binding to HSA are temperature dependant, and this may be due to the effect of temperature on the affinities of the HSA to MDP.

Test of other serum proteins binding to 99mTc-MDP

Since there are several proteins in the serum such as globlins, lipoproteins in addition to albumin, so there is a probability of binding ^{99m}Tc-MDP with one or more of these proteins rather than HSA after intra venious injection of ^{99m}Tc-MDP to the human blood, to make sure that only HSA was bound to 99mTc-MDP, α , β, γ-gloubuline was incubated with ^{99mT}c-MDP in viyro, at 37c and pH 7.4. fig (3.12) show that there is only one peak obtained when the radioactivity of each fraction collected from the column was plotted vs its corresponding raction number, there is no significant radioactivity appear in the first ten fractions, and there is one peak appeared between fraction 11 to 17 (the ^{99m}Tc-MDP position).

In order to identify the fractions containing the gloubulines, the absorbance of each fraction isolated by gel filteration was measured with uv-spectrophotometer at 280nm, there was asignificant absorbance happened in the fraction 4-8 which indicates that all gloubulins eluted in these fractions and there was no any interactions between ^{99m}Tc-MDP and these globulines. This results indicate that the ^{99m}Tc-MDP was bound only with HSA during the transport through the blood to reach its target organ he bone or skelecton.

Table (3.1): the specifically bound ^{99m}Tc-MDP to its binding protein (HSA) at optimum pH (7.4) and dfferent temperature

Temp c	Specifically bound of ^{99m}Tc-MDP at equilibrium ($\times 10^{-8}$m)
20	2.9
30	5.0
37	6.8
50	7.4

Table (3.2): Kd and Bmax values obtained from scatchard plot for the 99mTc-MDP binding with HSA at different temperature.

Temp c	Kd (nm)	Bmax (pmol/mg protein)
20	15.5	3.81
30	15.9	4.8
37	17.0	5.89
50	17.5	6.88

Table (3.3): Kd and Bmax values obtained from the double reciprocal lot for the 99mTc-MDP binding to purified HSA

Temp c	Kd ($\times 10^{-8}$M)	Bmax ($\times 10^{-8}$M)
20	5.14	1.50
30	6.72	1.59
37	8.84	1.76
50	11.16	1.92

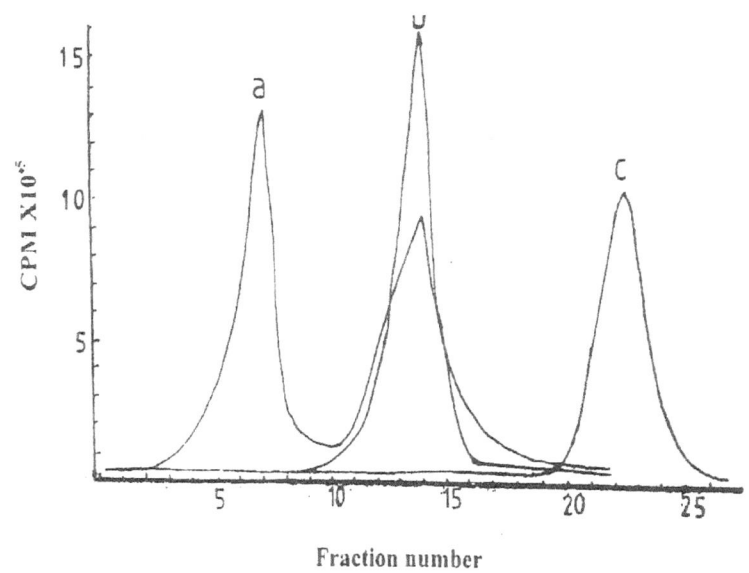

Fig (3.1) Separation of ^{99m}Tc , ^{99m}Tc-MDP and ^{99m}Tc-MDP- HSA complex using sephadex G-100 coloumn and pH 7.4 , (a) bound ^{99m}Tc-MDP- HSA complex , (b) ^{99m}Tc-MDP , (c) ^{99m}Tc only , all other details are explained in the text .

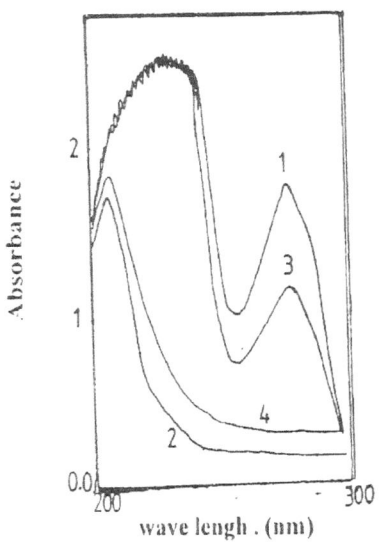

Fig (3.2) UV-spectra for four types of compounds , (1)HSA , (2) MDP , (3) ^{99m}Tc-MDP- HSA , (4) ^{99m}Tc-MDP , all details are explained in the

116

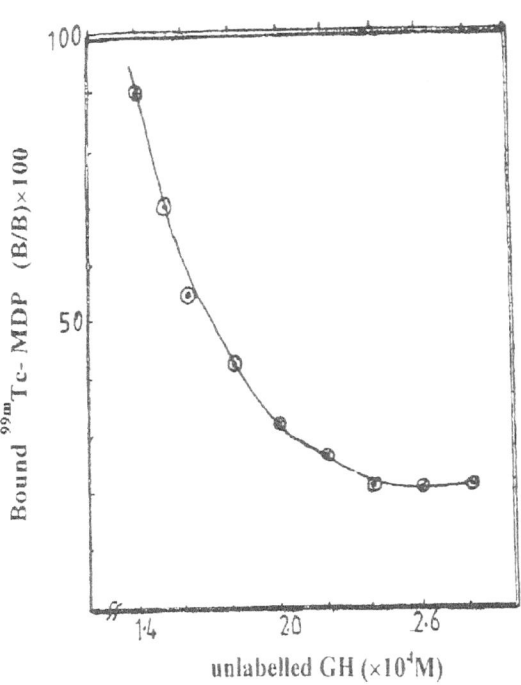

Fig (3.3) Non - specific binding determinition of ^{99m}Tc-MDP binding to purified HSA , all details are explained in the text .

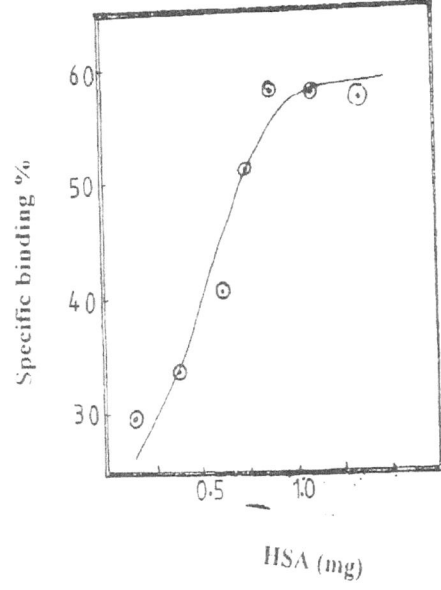

Fig (3.4) The effect of protein content on ^{99m}Tc-MDP binding to purified HSA . All details are explained in the text .

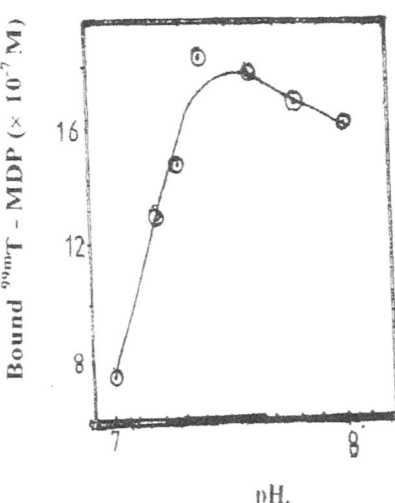

Fig (3.5) pH dependency of ^{99m}Tc-MDP binding to purified HSA , all details
are explained in the text .

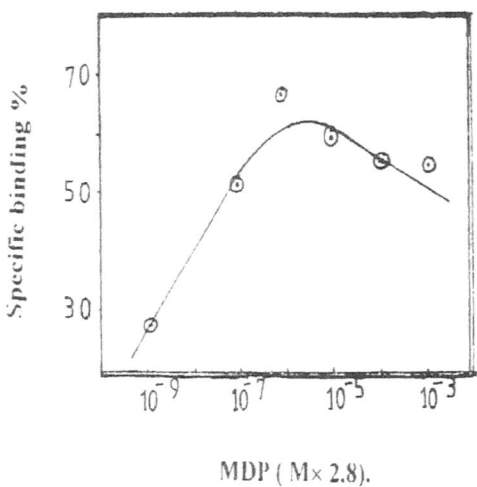

Fig (3.6) Binding of increasing concentrations of ^{99m}Tc-MDP to purified
HSA . All details are explained in the text .

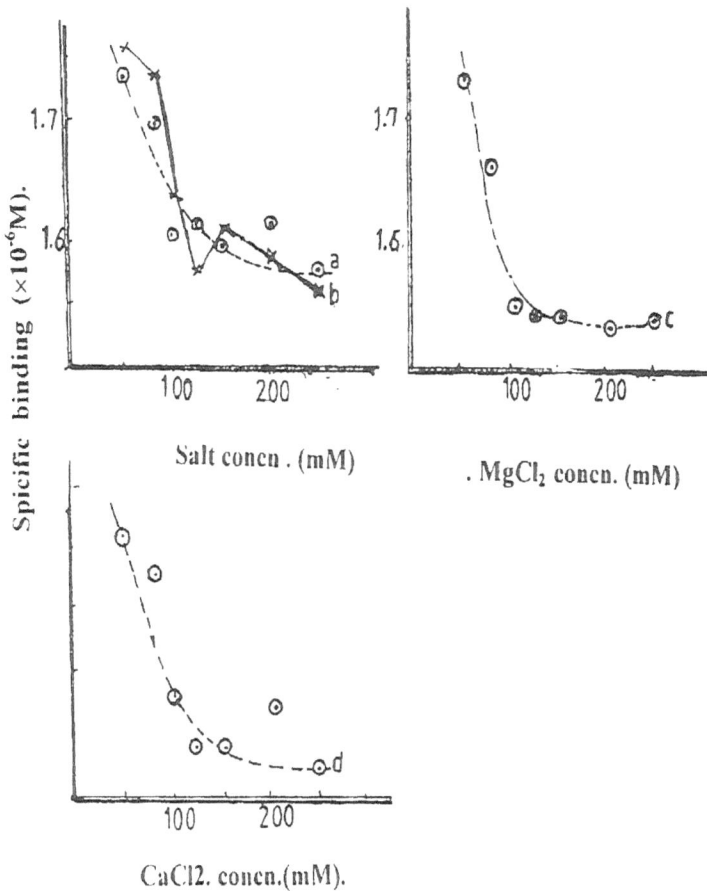

Fig (3.7) The effect of salt concentration on the ^{99m}Tc-MDP binding to HSA using (a) NaCl , (b) KCl , (c) MgCl$_2$, (d) CaCl$_2$ .All details are explained in the text.

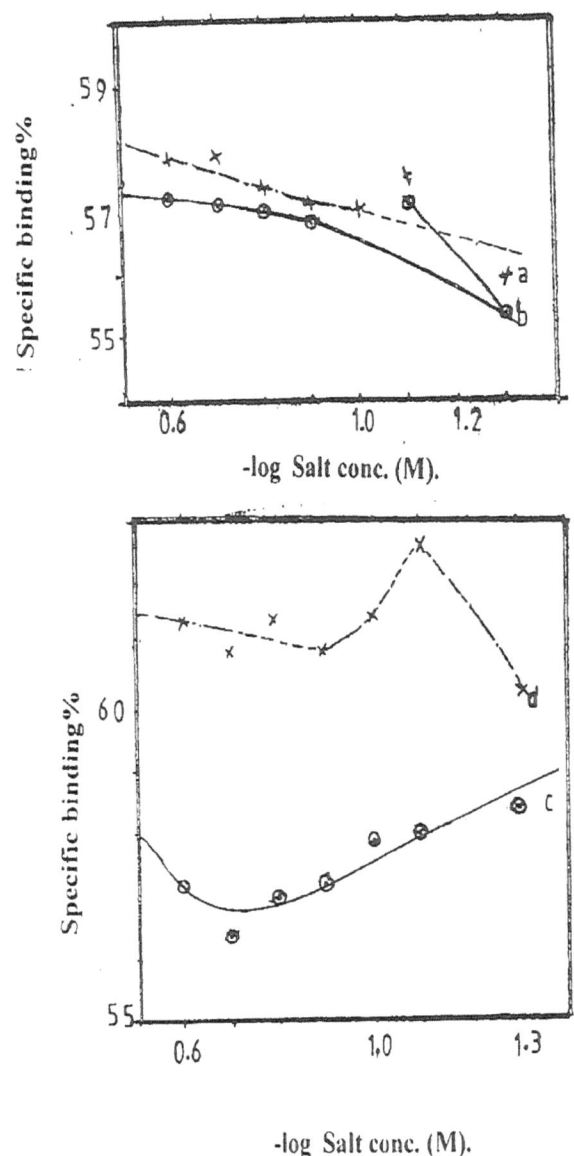

Fig(3.8):The effect of different concentration of (a)Na⁺;(b) k⁺: (c) Mg+2;(d) Ca+2 on the ^{99m}Tc-MDP binding to HSA . All deftails are outlined in the text .

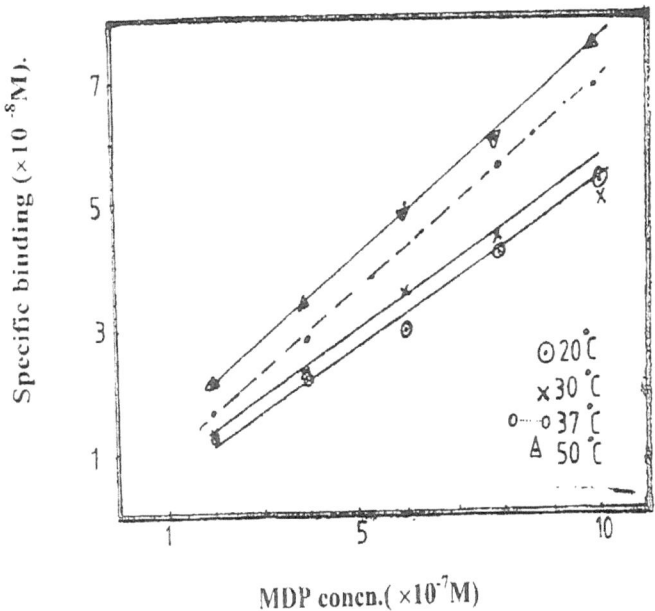

Fig(3.9):The relationshipe between specific binding and MDP concentration at equilibirium.All details are outline in the text

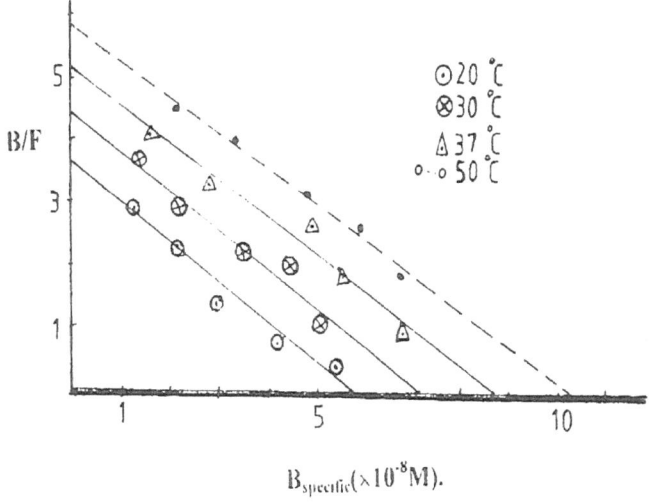

Fig(3.10):Scatchard plots of specific binding of ^{99m}Te-MDP to HSA at different temperature. All details are outline in the text.

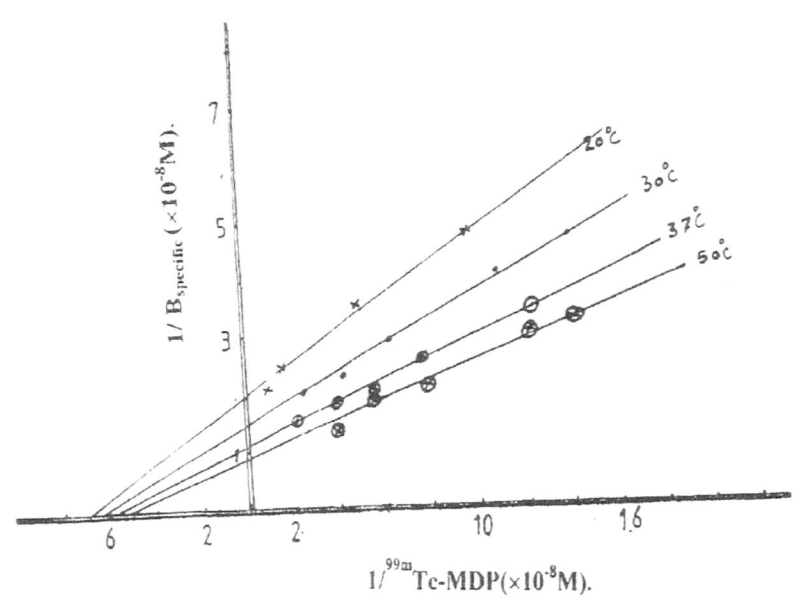

Fig(3.11):The double reciprocal plots of 99mTc - MDP binding to purified HSA at different temperature. All detail are explaind in the text.

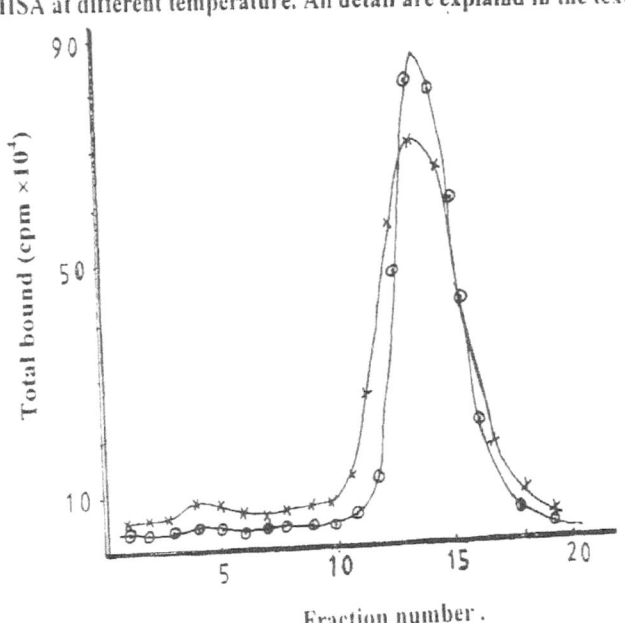

Fig(3.12):Elution profile for the reaction of 99mTc-MDP with γ gloubuline(x), and α, β-gloubuline⊙. All details are explained in the text.

Binding characteristics of ^{99}Tc-MDP to bone-binding protein (BBP).

SUMMARY

This chapter deals with the binding of ^{99m}Tc-MDP to the bone binding protein (BBP). The specificity of ^{99m}Tc-MDP binding to the (BBP) was examined, the results show that the non specific binding was 8-12% of the total binding. The effect of mono and divalent chloride salts were also examined.

The optimum pH for the binding was 7.4, the most suitable amounts of MDP concentration to give maximum binding was 2.8×10^{-6}m. the association constant Ka and maximum binding capacities Bmax of ^{99m}Tc-MDP to its binding sites was determined from scatchard plots. The results revealed that Ka and Bmax values were temperature dependent.

INTRODUCTION

Bone has an abundant noncollagenous protein which contain the vitamin K-dependant amino acid, γ-carboxyglutamic acid (247, 248). This amino acid has been identified in bovine prothrombin, gama-carboxyglutamic acid (Gla), is synthesized from glutamic acid residues in apost translation enzymatic reaction with an absolute requirement for vitamin K and bicarbonate (249) as shown in this reaction:

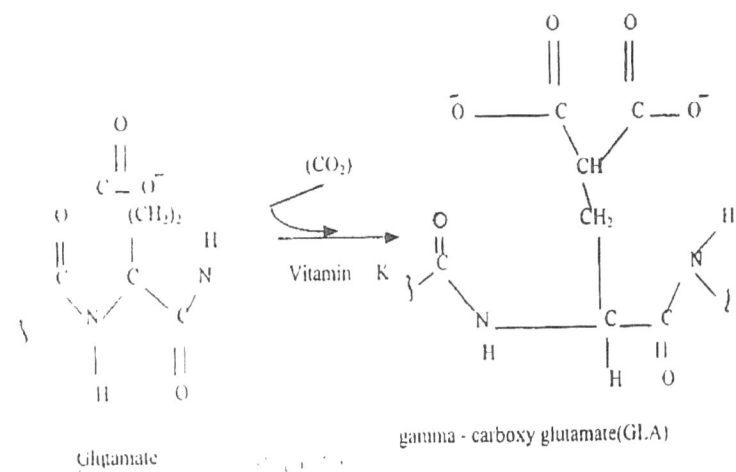

Fig(4.1)Post-translational carboxylation of glutamic acid to give gamm-carboxyglutamic acid.

Gla-protein is secreted by bone cells into plasma and other extracellular fluids and subsequently accumulates in bone by binding to mineral (250). Some studies have shown that the biosythesis of gla protein is dramatically stimulated by physiological level of 1, 25-dihydroxyvitamin D3 (250), this suggests that the protein may mediate an aspect of the action of vitamin D on bone (251).

Paul A.P. et al (252) have characterized the gamma-arboxyglumatic acid contaning protein from bovine bone, they found that the bovine-Gla stoichiometry of bone Gla protein (BGP) per crystal and that the bovine Gla protein is a protent inhibitor of hydroxyapatite crystallixation another author (253) clamed that Gla protein binds strongly and reversible to hydroxyapatite, it will not nind to amorphous calcium phosphate. It has been postulated that he protein may be involved in establishing or maintaining Ca_{+2} and toal bone mineral homeostasis perhaps serving a hormonal function (254). In vitro studies have shown that the alf bone Gla protein is an effective inhibitor of the precipitation of calcium phosphate from saturated solution (225), while it has low affinity for Ca_{+2} (Kd=3mm) for three binding sites (256). The isolation and complete amino acid sequence of the human bone Gla protein have been studied (252).

In fetal human bone, the level of bone Gla protein is one gram of BGP per one mole of bone PO4, rise from 5% of the adult level at 10 week gestational age of the adult level at 15 week (257). The covalent structure has been determined for BGP isolated from calf, wordfish, human, chiken, and monky bone (252, 257, 258) direct comparison of these structures reveals a remarkable degree of conservation over evaluationary time (109).

Our aim in this chapter is to establish the parameters which effect the ^{99m}Tc-MDP binding to the BBP , and to find the maximum binding was obtained.

4.1 HUMAN BONE COLLECTION AND PREPARATION

1- malignant tumour of human bone ovtained from alshahed-addnan hospital-baghdad were taken from patients (18-30 yrs age) and examined histologically and in each case malignant tunour was confirmed,

2- bone specimens were immediately immersed in ice-cold saline and then washed with phosphate buffer pH 7.4, cleaned from adhering connective tissue and ground into segments of approximately one mm in longest dimension, and washed several time with cold phosphate buffer (4c), dried and kept at-20c until homogenization.

3- the frozen sample were homogenized in 50 mm phosphate buffer pH7.4, the ratio of the bone tissue to the buffer solution was 1:4 (w/v) using tenbroeck ground-glass homogenizer to prepare the homogenate.

4- the bone tissue homogenate was filtered through tem layers of the nylon gauze, then centrifuged at 3000rpm for 25 minutes in order to precipitate the remaining intact cells. The supernatant was used throughout our study and stored at-20c till using.

4.3 PURIFICATION OF BONE PROTEIN

4.2.1 preparation and packing of the column:

1- the gel was prepared by swelling 40 mg of sephadox-G100 in 450ml of 50 mm phosphate buffer pH 7.4 for 24 hours at room temperature (about 30c) then stored at 4c to equilibrated it with the buffer.

2- the suspension was carefully mixed before pouring into vertical column (with diameter of 2cm) contaning eluent buffer. After the gel has setted, the column outlet was opened. Packing was continued until the gel reached stable bed height (100cm) then the coumn was equilibrated with 50mm phosphate buffer pH 7.4 with rate of 10ml per hour, then the sample was applied to the surface of the gel carefully to separate the bone protein.

4.2.2 purification of bone protein:

1- 100μl EDTA solution (0.5m) was added to 1ml supernatant which is prepared in experiment (4.1) with stirring, after 1h the solution was applied to the surface of the sephadex G-100 column prepared in section 4.2.1 equilibrated with buffer pH 7.4.

2- the sample was eluted using the same buffer with flow eate of 12ml/h, and fraction volume each of 2ml were collected.

3- the spectrum of each fraction was measured using uv-vis spectrophotometer. The absorbance at 280 nm of each fraction was plotted against its corresponding fraction number.

4.2.3 protein determination:

Protein concentration in the bone sample was determined by lowry et al (259) method using human serum albumin as the internal standard (fig 4.2), the supernatant prepared in experiment (4.1) was used for this purpose.

4.3 PRELIMINARY TEST FOR THE BINDING OF ^{99m}Tc-MDP TO BONE HOMOGENATE

The binding of ^{99m}Tc-MDP to bone homogenate was primarily checked as following:

1- 100µl bone homogenate (protein concentration 18µg/ml) was incubated with 100µl ^{99m}Tc-MDP (2.8×10^{-6}m) at 30°c for 30 minutes, the final volume was completed up to 500µl with phosphate buffer pH 7.4.

2- the sample was applied to the surface of sephadex G-100 gel filteration column (1.0x30cm) equilibrated with 50mm phosphate buffer pH 7.4. Elution was carried out using the same buffer to separate bound ^{99m}Tc-MDP-bone protein complex from free ^{99m}Tc-MDP with flow rate of 12ml/h, and fraction volumes of 2ml.

3- radioactivity of each fraction tube in cpm was counted using γ-counter.

4- the steps from 1-3 were repeated with the addition of 25μl of unlabelled GH with concentrations ranging from 1.4×10^{-4}-2.8×10^{-4}m).

Calculation :

1- total binding (TB) represents the amount of radioactivity bound to the BBP fraction (expressed in counts per minutes, cpm) in the absence of unlabelled GH.

2- the radioactivity of the BBP fractions after the maximum displacement of the ^{99m}Tc-MDP by excess amounts of unlabelled GH is reffered to as nonspecific binding (NB).

3- Specific binding (SB) is the difference between radioactivity (cpm) bound of the paraticulate fraction in the absence of excess unlabelled GH (TB) and that bound in its presence (NB).

SB (cpm) = TB (cpm) –NB (cpm)

4- SB% can be obtained from the following formula:

$$SB\% = \frac{SB(cpm)}{total\ count(cpm)of\ ^{99m}Tc\text{-}MDP\ used\ in\ incubation\ tube(\ Tc\ )} \times 100$$

Solutions and preparation of sephadex G100 column:

1- 5ml saline was added to kit vial prepared in section 3.2, then 1ml of the solution was diluted to 10ml with phosphate buffer pH7.4 to get 2.8×10^{-6}m concentration of MDP.

2- ^{99m}Tc-MDP was prepared by the addition of 10μl ^{99m}Tc to the MDP solution in step (1).

3- Unlabelled gloucoheptonate (GH) solutions were prepared by serial dilution of 0.28mm GH solution, using phosphate buffer pH7.4.

4- Preparation and packing the gel:

(a) the gel was prepared by swelling 10mg of sephdox G-100 in 100ml phosphate buffer pH 7.4, for 24 hpurs at 30c then stored at 4c to equilibrate it with the buffer.

(b) The suspension was carefully mixed before pouring into vertical columns (with diameter of 1.0cm) containing eluent buffer. After the gel has settled, the column outlet was opened. Packing was continued until the gel reached astable bed height (30.0cm) then column was equilibrated with phosphate buffer pH 7.4, with flow rate of 12ml/h then the sample (500μl) was applied to the surface of the gel carefully to separate bound ^{99m}Tc-MDP-complex from the free ^{99m}Tc-MDP. Elution was carried out using the same buffer of equilibration with flow rate of 12ml/h and fraction volume of 2ml.

4.3.1 effect of pH on the binding of ^{99m}Tc-MDP to its binding protiem in bone homogenate:

1- 100μl of bone homogenate was incubated with 100μl ^{99m}Tc-MDP (2.8×10^{-6}m) at 30c (room temperature) for 30 minutes at different pH ranging from (7.0, 7.2, 7.4, 7.6, 7.8, 8.0) phosphate buffer, the final volume was 500μl for all samples using the same buffer.

2- the steps 2-4 of the experiment 4.3 were followed.

Calculations:

1- the same mathematical formula mentioned in experiment 4.3 was used to calculate specific binding SB%.

2- Specific binding SB% was converted to bound ^{99m}Tc-MDP in molarity according to the following formula:

Specifically bound = SB% x total ^{99m}Tc-MDP concn.in incubation ^{99m}Tc-MDP in (molar)   media in (M)

3- Specifically bound ^{99m}Tc-MDP in molar was plotted vs. their corresponding pH.

4.3.2 effect of monovalent and divalent salts on binding of ^{99m}Tc-MDP to bone homogenate:

4.3.2.1 effect of monovalent salts on binding of ^{99m}Tc-MDP to bone homogenate:

1- 100μl of bone homogenate was incubated with 100μl ^{99m}Tc-MDP (2.8×10^{-6}m) at 37c and pH 7.4 for 30 minutes in presence of different concentrations of NaCI or KCI (from 50-250mm).

2- steps (2-4) of experiment (4.3) were repeated.

Calculation:

1- specifiv binding % of each salt concentration was determined as in experiment (4.3).

132

2- the amount of specifically bound ^{99m}Tc-MDP in molar of each salt concentration was determined as in experiment (4.3.1).

3- the amounts of specifically bound ^{99m}Tc-MDP in molar were plotted vs the salts concentration in the incubation media.

4.3.2.2 effect of divalent salts on ^{99m}Tc-MDP binding to bone homogenate:

1- 100μl of bone homogenate was incubated with 100μl ^{99m}Tc-MDP (2.8×10^{-6}m) at 30°c and pH 7.4 for 30minutes in presence of different concentrations from 50mm to 250mm of MgCl$_2$ or CaCl$_2$.

2- steps 2-4 of experiment 4.3 were repeated.

Calculation:

The same mathematical formula mentioned in experiment 4.3.2.1 were followed

Solution:

1- stock KCI (1M) : 7.45g of KCI was dissolved and made up to 100ml with phosphate buffer pH 7.4 from this solution all the other different concentrations were prepared by serial dilution.

2- Stock NaCI (M): 5.85g of NaCI was dissolved and made up to 100ml with phosphate buffer pH 7.4 from this solution all the other different concentrations were prepared by serial dilution.

3- Stock MgCl2 (1M): 20.33g of $MgCl_2.6H_2O$ was dissolved and made up to 100ml by the same buffer.

4- Stock $CaCl_2$ (1M) : 11.1g of $CaCl_2$ was dissolved and made up to 199ml by the same buffer.

4.3.2.3 choice of the most appropriate amount of MDP for the binding of ^{99m}Tc-MDP with bone homogenate:

1- 100μl of bone homogenate was added to 100μl of each MDP concentration ranging from 2.8×10^{-3} to 2.8×10^{-9} molar. The total volume was completed to 500μl with phosphate buffer pH 7.4 and incubated for 30 minutes at room temperature (30°c).

2- the steps (2-4) of experiment (4.3) were followed.

Calculation:

1- specific binding % of each MDP concentration was determined as in experiment (4.3).

2- the specific binding (SB%) of ^{99m}Tc-MDP of each concentration was plotted vs. MDP concentration in incubation media.

4.4 SATURATION EXPERIMENT AND SCATCHARD ANALYSIS

1- 100µl of bone homogenate was incubated with increasing amount of ^{99m}Tc-MDP from (0.20 to 1.0 µM) in afinal volume of 500µl.

2- aparallel set of assay tubes were used to determine non-specific binding as outlined in the previous experiments.

3- all the tubes were incubated at 37°c and pH 7.4 for 30 minutes.

4- the step (2-4) in experiment (4.3) were performed in different temperatures (20, 30 and 50°c).

Calculation:

1- the values of ^{99m}Tc-MDP bound specifically in molar (Bspecific) ere calculated using the following formula:

$$B_{specific} = \frac{total\ binding(\ TB\ ) - nonspecific\ binding(\ NB\ )}{total\ count(\ TC\ )} \times conc\ of\ ^{99m}Tc - MDP\ in\ molar$$

2- Bspecific was plotted vs concentration of ^{99m}Tc-MDP (M) used in incubation medium.

3- The plot of B/F values versus the value of Bspecific gives a linear relationship from the values of the affinity constant (Ka) and the total binding site numbers, maximum binding capacitites (Bmax) were calculated according to the following relation:

$$B/F = (1/Kd)\ (Bmax-Bspecific)$$

135

Where : B is the bound radioactivity (cpm) which represents the ^{99m}Tc-MDP binding bone homogenate complex. F is the radioactivity (cpm) which represents non bound ^{99m}Tc-MDP.

F= total count (cpm)-bound radioactivity (B)

4- Kd and Bmax value were also obtained from the double reciprocal plot of data getting from scatchard plots, using the follwing formula:

1/Bspecific = (Kd/Bmax x 1/(F) + 1/Bmax

1/Bspecific values were pletted vs 1/(F)

1/Kd values was obtained from intercept on abscissa.

1/Bmax value was obtained from intercept on ordinate.

4.5 BINDING OF ^{99m}Tc-MDP TO PURIFIELD BONE PROTEIN

1- 100μl of purified bone protein (18.2μg/ml) was added to 100μl of each MDP concentration ranging from 2.0×10^{-7} to 14×10^{-7} molar the total volume was completed to 500μl using phosphate buffer pH 7.4 and incubated for 30 minutes at 37°c.

2- the steps (2-4) of experiment (4.3) were repeated.

Calculation:

1- the same mathematical formulas mentioned in experiment (4.3) were followed to calculate the percent of specific binding of ^{99m}Tc-MDP to bone protein.

Solutions:

The same as mentionaed in experiment (4.3).

The amount of ^{99m}Tc used:

Almost the same volume of radioactive ^{99m}Tc (10µl) was used in all experiments in this work, the amount of ^{99m}Tc in (pg) was calculated according to the following (1):

(1) 1mci=3.7x107 dps

(2) 1 (mci) x 3.7 x 107 (dps) x 6 (h) x 60 (s/h) x 1.443=1.922x10^{10} disintigration where: the average life is 1.443 times the half-life.

(3) nimber of atoms per gram atimic weight:

1mci ^{99m}Tc = 1.922x1010 atoms =

$$= 3.159 \times 10\text{-}12g$$

Or 1mci ^{99m}Tc = 3.159 peco gram

(4) 10µci ^{99m}Tc= 0.03159 pg ^{99m}Tc

$$= 31.59 \text{ femto gram}$$

RESULTS AND DISCUTSION

Human bone preparation:

The bone samples were cleaned from any adhering connective tissue to prevent contamination with other protein rather than that of bone homogenization of the samples were carried out in acold medium (4˚c) to avoid protein denaturation (260, 261). The filteration of the bone homogenate through ten layers of the nylon gauze was used to remove any suspened pieces of unhomogenized fragments, while centrifugation of the homogenate at 3600 rpm removed the unruptured cells and other bone matrix, from the supernatant (262) which could be used as the bone homogenate source in this chapter.

Purification of bone protein:

One of the most remarkable facts about bone γ-carboxy glutaic acid protein (BGP) is its abundance, it comprises 1-2% of the protein in a typical vertebrate bone (245, 247, 249). Two general procedures have been devised for isolating BGP from bone (252), both entail first grinding dried cortical bone to a consistency of coarse sand in a blender or for large-scale a mill. In one extraction method, 0.5 M-EDTA, pH 7.4 was used to demenerlized the extract , purification of BGP from the extract is then achieved by gel filteration over sephadex G100 (247). The second procedure was developed to permit the isolation of BGP in the presence of endogenous proteases. BGP is extracted by demineralization of bone with 10 parts by weight of 10% formic acid and then gel-filteration over asephacryl (255).

Our method depend on the procedure of price et al. (247) after gel filtration on sephadex G100 using phosphate buffer pH7.4, the absorbace of each fraction was measured at (280nm), three absorption peak were obtained fig (4.1). the second peak represent the Gla protein. The identification of Gla protein depend on the methods that puplished by other authors (263,264).

The amount of protein I the fractions of 2nd peak was determined according to lowry method using HSA as standard as shown in fig (4.2), the result indicate that the amount of Gla protein is 18.2ug/1g dry bone powder.

Preliminary test for the bindnig of ^{99m}Tc-MDP to bone homogenate :

The homogenate containing bone proeins and mierals fraction was used as the bone source to investigate how the ^{99m}Tc-MDP binding was carried out. After 30 minutes of incubation at 30c the bound ^{99m}Tc-MDP was separated by gel filteration chromatograph using sephadex G100 column (1x30cm). the bond ^{99m}Tc-MDP was observed in fractions 4-9 whereas the non bound was observed in fractions 12-17 in the same pattern of ^{99m}Tc-MDP elution as in fig (4.3).

The specificity of the binding was investigated by introducing different concentrations of unlabelled GH into incubation medium. The concentration of unlabelled GH (molar) which was necessary to cause a maximum displacement of the ^{99m}Tc-MDP, equal 100 times that of ^{99m}Tc-MDP concentration. About 88-90% of the bound ^{99m}Tc-MDP was displaced from its binding proteins in bone homogenate, hence the non specific binding was 8-12%. The amount of non specificity remaining constant whatever the concentrations of the unlabelled GH used fig (4.4). Watkins and white found that the ^{125}I-CaM binding to islet sectetion granules, the amount of ^{125}I-CaM bound was reduced by 92% on the addition of excess (200nm) unlabelled.

The effect of pH on the ^{99m}Tc-MDP binding to its binding sites in bone homogenate:

Fig (4.5) show the effect of incrasing pH from 7.0 to 8.0 on the binding of ^{99m}Tc-MDP to its binding protein in bone homogenate. Maximum value of the specific binding occurred at pH 7.4 (exhibits a narrow pH optimum). The results indicate that in general, binding was pH-dependent and the shift in the pH of environment may affect the properties of the particulate involved in binding.

The pH dependence of the binding indicates that protonation deprotonation reactions are important to the energetics of ^{99m}Tc-MDP-bone homogenate, the destabilization of the complex at low pH may be due to increase in the dissociation rate of the complex formed. So the choice of appropriate pH and reductive environment may be maintained (265, 266).

Our results almost on line with that found by garnett et al (267). The most important variables affecting the reative abundance of the various components of a ^{99m}Tc-bone scanning agent are the pH (132, 268-270).

Effect of MDP concentration on the binding t the bone homogenate:

When ^{99m}Tc-MDP was added to the bone homogenate solution, and sparation was accomplished on the gel chromatography, the results show that the total binding increased with incrasing MDP concentration until the concentration of 2.8×10^{-6}M, then equilibrium was took place and saturation was reached. Tis results shown in fig (4.6), from these data we can not conclude whether ^{99m}Tc-MDP attached to the matrix or to the bone proteins , but in general the total binding in case of bone homogenate sample is less than that with albumin lone or with bone protein extract there are many papers clamid that ^{99m}Tc-MDP was adsorbed on the hydroxyapatite of the bone , avery good review on this subject was published by deligny et al. (121), the influence of various species that occur in the bone flid and of some other variables on the assorption of ^{99m}Tc-MDP on hydroxyaptite have been studied (271). Athrough discussion on the mineral phase of bone and of the interaction of diphosphonates with it, and the action of various chemical species that adsorb on the crystal surfaces of synthetic and biological apatites and which poson their formation and growth (272). Arapid exchange between bone mineral and the extra-celluar fluid in bone is the basis for the short-term fixation of a bone-seeking eadionuclide in bone (273). There is stronge evidence that any bone uptake of a bone seeking agent is related to bone formation (273, 275),and that uptake in the calcifying bone matrix is under the control of bone cells (276). The chemical structure of the iphosphonate is well known, but not that of the complexes formed with reduced [99mTc] (277). It has been shown once ore that the biodistribution of [99mTc]-diphosphonate complexes is related to the chemical properties of the diphosphonate in use one major factor is the compkex stability between reduced [99mTc] and the diphosphnate (278).

Effect of monovalent and divalent salts on the binding of [99mTc]-MDP to the bone homogenate:

Fig (7.4) A and B show the effect of monovalent salt (NaCI and KCI) and divalent sat ($CaCI_2$ and MgI_2) respectively from the results there is no significant effect on the binding of [99mTc]-MDP to the bone homogenate, there is slightly decrease ith $MgCI_2$, and small increasing of the binding in presence of 120 mm $CaCI_2$. the conclusion from this data indicate that there is no any interaction between the ions of these salts with the active site or binding sites at this pH (7.4), also there is no any competition between diphosphonate anion and chloride anions. Huigen et al (274) ave mentioned that the adsorption of [99mTc]-MDP to bone matrix was decreased in the prescense of Mg_{+2} also the anionsHCO3 and SO4 do not show large effects, while asmall positive effect is found with Ca_{+2} and large decrease in presence of Sn_{+2}. Pinkerton et al (279) have mentioned that passage occurs by diffusion, it was established that the rate of diffusion through capillary walls does not depend on the charge of the diffusing particle.

Saturation experiments:

Fig (4.8) represent the saturation curves and effect of increasing ^{99m}Tc-MDP concentrations on the binding to bone homogenate at 20, 30, 37 and 50c. the result indicated that the amount of ^{99m}Tc-MDP bound to its binding sites increased with temperature and depend on the MDP concentration, reaching the equilibrium around 1.2×10^{-6}M ^{99m}Tc-MDP. Increasing the temperature from 20c to 50c rised the specific binding of ^{99m}Tc-MDP about 1.3 fold.

Determination of affinity constant (Ka) and maximum binding capacity:

Fig (4.9) represent the scatchard plots for binding of ^{99m}Tc-MDP to bone homogenate at different temperatures from which the dissociation constants (K_d) and maximum binding capacities (Bmax) were determined table (4.1).

Increasing temperature from 20c to 50c Bmax was increased 1.699 folds, this results indiat that the Bmax is atemperature dependant, while Kd is not. The results indicate that the complex formed between ^{99m}Tc-MDP with bone is stable where Ka equal to 8.06×10^{6}, 9.09×10^{6}, 8.55×10^{6} and 8.85×10^{6} ,olar at

20, 30, 37 and 50˚c respectively, and it is temperature independent, this is may be due affinity of bone proteins or bone matrix to bind ^{99m}Tc-MDP directly and strangly with out any additive, this is good phenomena, and give good picture of bone after intravenous injection of ^{99m}Tc-MDP to the body.

Effect of reaction time and temperature on the binding of ^{99m}Tc-MDP with bone homogenate:

In general the amount of binding ^{99m}Tc-MDP at pH7.4 phosphate buffer, increased with incrasing the incubation time reaching maximum value then decreased with time. There is no significant effect of temperature on the maximum binding in the range 30c to 60c. fig (4.11) show that the specific binding at 20c appeared after 45 minutes of incubation time, and there is no change in the specific binding, this indicate that dissociation of ^{99m}Tc-MDP bone complex is very small i.e the complex formed is stable at that temperature after two hours f incubation time.

At 30 and 37c the equilibrium reached after 30 minutes incubation time, and after 20 minutes at 50˚c and 60˚c, the decreases of the specific binding with incrasing incubation time at high temperature (more than 30c) may be due to the dissociation of the complex formed between ^{99m}Tc-MDP and bone homogenate. Garnett et al (267) have mentioned that the temperature have minimal effect on ^{99m}Tc-diphosphonate stability. Hughes et al (280) was published that the median

144

residence time in the perivascular and bone fluids is about 16 minutes, and during this time a limited amount of hydrolysis may occur. As the size of the hydrolysis products of bone scanning agent is probably much larger than of its original components (by coprecipitation and adsorption phenomena) diffusion through the pores between the bone lining cell will be slow and so adsorption on the hydroxyapatite crystals will be hampered (281, 282).

Binding of ^{99m}Tc-MDP to purified bone protein:

Fig (4.12) show the specific binding (in m mole) of ^{99m}Tc-MDP to the purified bone protein which is named GBP, (247) the results indicate that the specific binding inreases with increasing MDP concentration, reach amaximum value at ^{99m}Tc-MDP concentration of ^{99m}Tc-MDP with bone homogenate.

The results indicate that ^{99m}Tc-MDP has good affinity to the binding sites of BGP , means that the ^{99m}Tc-MDP did not adsorbed completely on the hydroxyaptite, but it binds to BGP but not to hydroxyapatite. The Gla protein binds strongly and reversibly to hydroxyapatite and half of the protein is adsorbed at acrystal concentration of 0.4 mg/ml (247). The Kd value I 0.5μM (257), while scatchard plot of Ca_{+2} binding to BGP shows three Ca_{+2} binding sites with an average dissociation constant of 3μM, BGP has less affinity to bind amorphous calcium phosphate, (247) and has a good ability to inhibit hydroxyapatie precipitation from supersaturated solutions. The presence of BGP in serum and the (250) elevated levels of serum BGP found in patients with metabolic bone diseases characterized by high bone turnover (258) suggest that the informational function of BGP may involve the regulation of bone turnover. These obsevations support our conclution that ^{99m}Tc-MDP was bind BGP but not to hydroxyapatite as mentioned y many authors (247, 258).

Table (4.1): Kd and Bmax value of ^{99m}Tc-MDP binding to its binding proteins in bone homogenate at different temperature determined from scatchard plot.

Temp c	Kd (μm)	Bmax (μm) 10^{-4}
20	0.124	4.63
30	0.110	5.34
37	0.117	6.90
50	0.113	7.87

Table (4.2): Kd and Bmax values of ^{99m}Tc-MDP binding to its binding proteins in bone homogenate at different temperature determined from double reciprocal

Temp c	Kd (10^{-7}m)	Bmax (10^{-7}m)
30	2.03	5.81
37	1.35	7.20
50	1.64	8.01

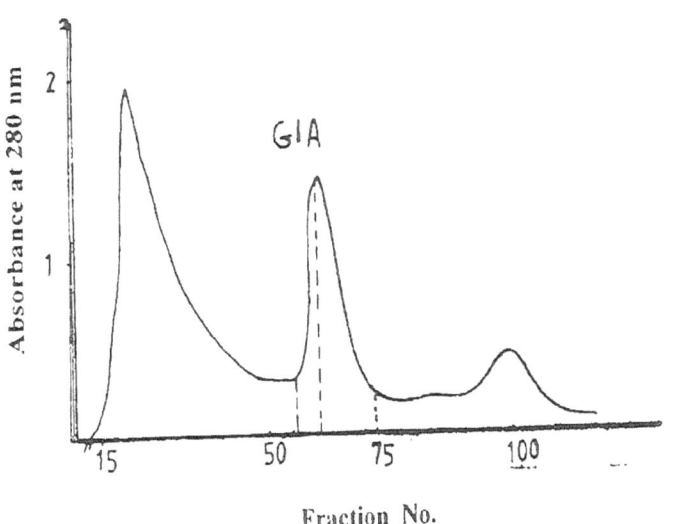

Fig(4.1):Gel filtration of human bone extract on (2×100 cm) column of
sephadex G- 100 with phosphate buffer pH 7.4 , 2ml per fraction
.All details are explaind in the text .

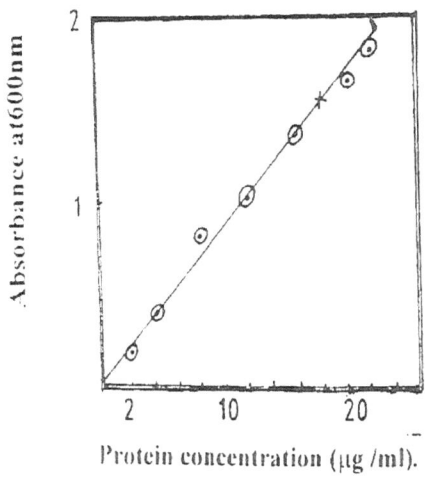

Fig(4.2):Standard curve of protein determination by Lowry method (using
HSA as standard) for Gla protein .

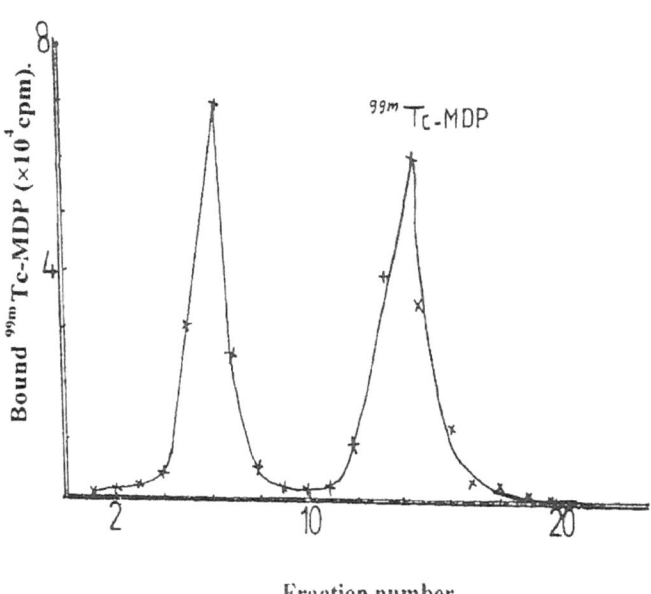

Fig(4.3): The elution profiles of the ^{99m}Tc-MDP-bone homogenate complex, from sephadex G-100 column. All details are explaind in the text .

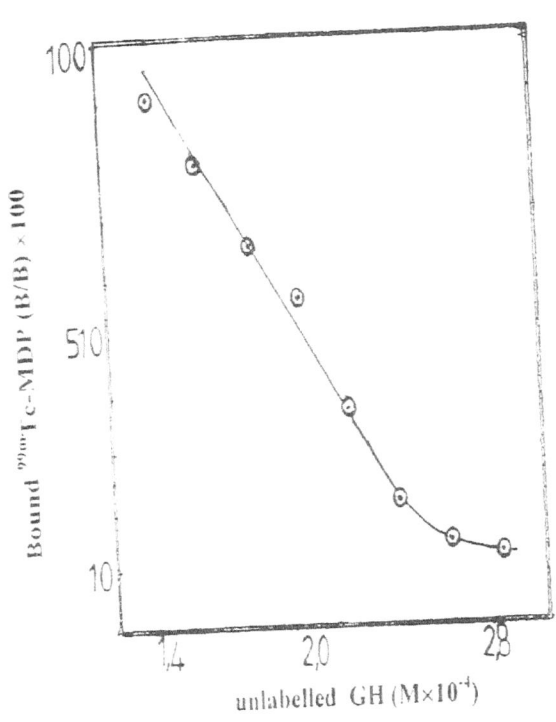

Fig(4.4):Non-specific binding determination of 99mTc-MDP binding to
bone homogenate .All details are explaind in the text .

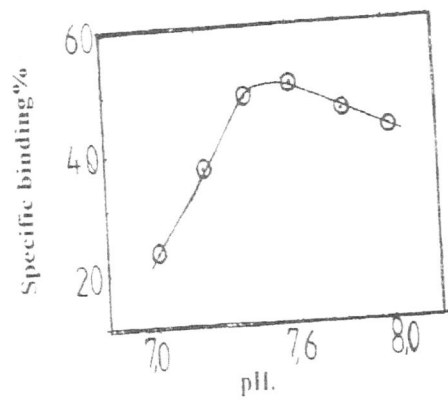

Fig(4.5):pH dependant of 99mTc-binding to bone homogenate. All detail
are explaind in the text .

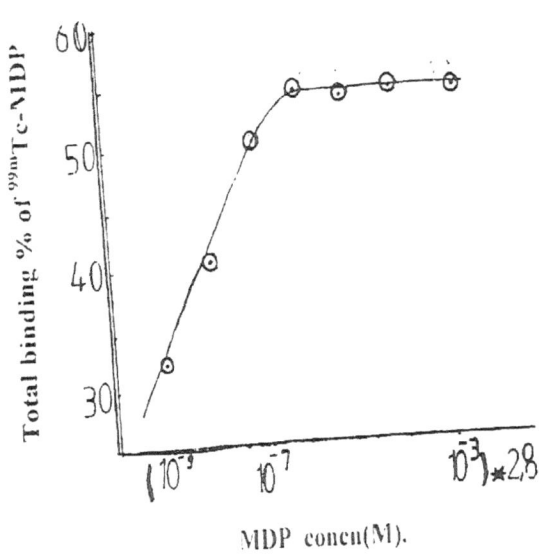

Fig(4.6): The effect of MDP concentration (molar)on the binding with the bone homogenate . All details are explaind in the text .

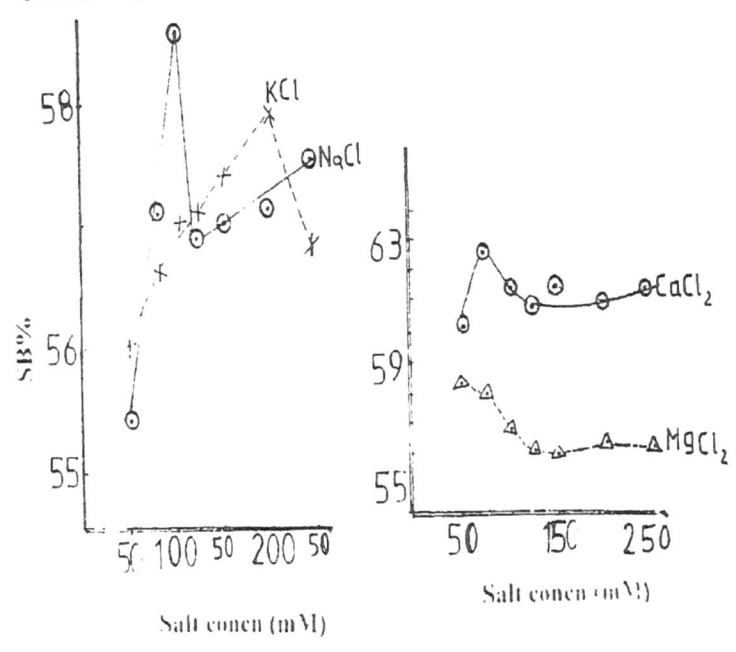

Fig(4.7): The effect of salt concentration on the ^{99m}Tc-MDP binding to the homogenate . All details are explained in the text.

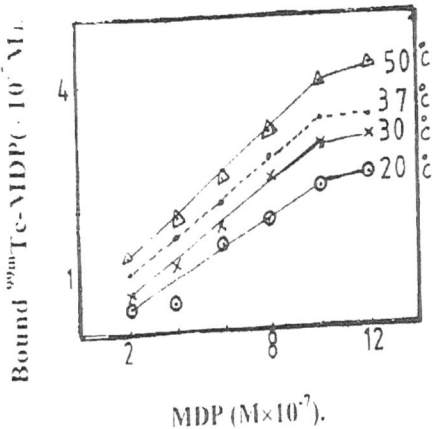

Fig(4.8):Binding of increasing concentration of 99mTc- MDP to bone
homogenate at 20,30,37and 50°c and pH 7.4 All details are
explaind in the text .

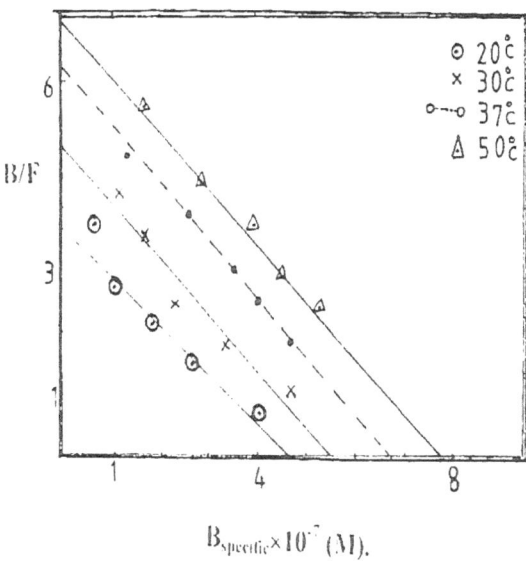

Fig(4.9):Seatchard plots of ^{99m}Tc-MDP binding to bone homogenare at
different temp. All details are explained in the text .

151

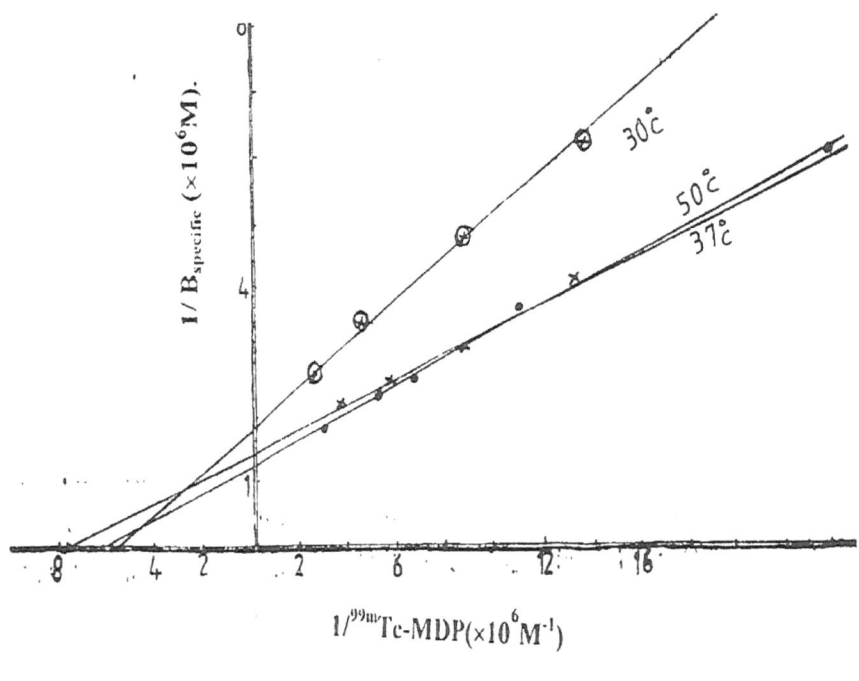

Fig(4.10):The double reciprocal plots of ^{99m}Tc -MDP binding to bone homogenate at different temp.(i.e. 30, 73 and 50°c).

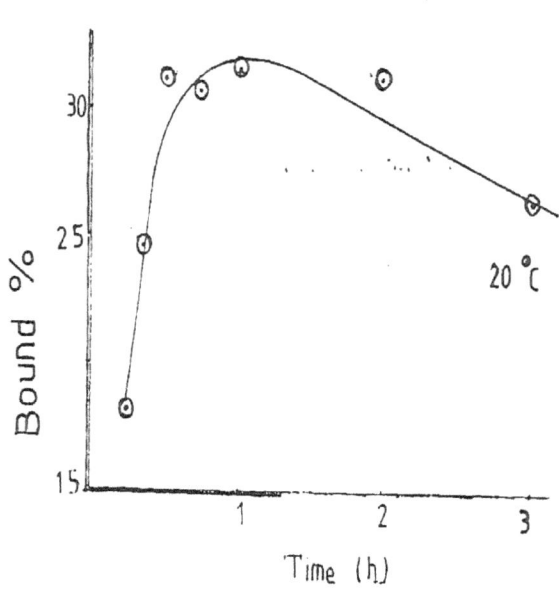

Fig(4.11):Effect of reaction temp. and time on binding study .

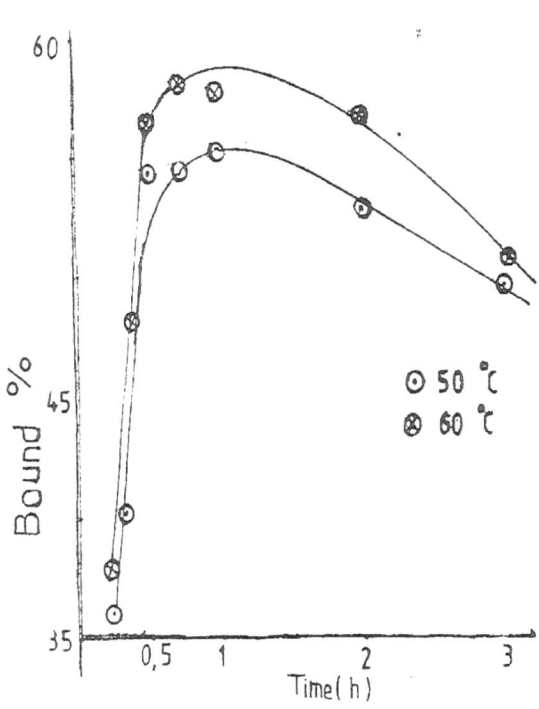

Fig (4.11)-continue.

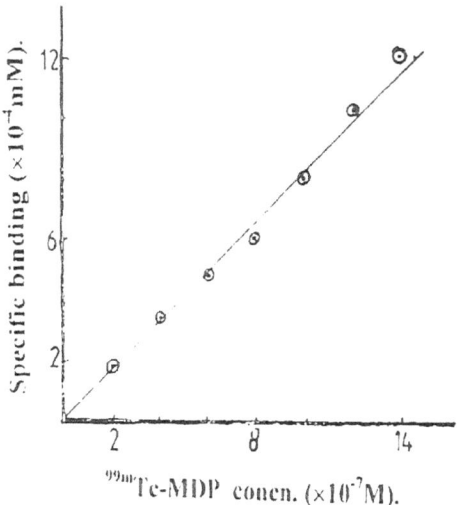

Fig(4.12):Binding of increasing amount of ^{99m}Tc - MDP to purified bone protein(BGP) at 37°c. All detail are outline in the text.

153

Kinetic and thermodynamic studies on ^{99}Tc-MDP binding to HSA and BBP.

SUMMARY

Kinetic and thermodynamic parameters associated with the binding of ^{99m}Tc-MDP to purified HSA and BBP from bone homogenate were inventigated. In the case of HSA, when the reaction temperature was increased from 20 to 37°c, the association rate constant K+1 was decrased by appyoximately 4.5% and 12.06% incase of BBP of bone homogenate. The hill plot data revealed that there was no copperativity between the MDP-binding sites in both HSA and bone homogenate.

The van't hoff plot demonstrated alinear relationship between in Ka and 1/T, the parameters for the equilibrium reactions described by ΔG, ΔH and ΔS were determined. Arrhenius plot indicated that there was a linear relationship between log K+1 or log Bmax and 1/T from which the transition state thermodynamic parameters for the formation of the ^{99m}Tc-MDP-HSA complex or ^{99m}Tc-MDP-bone complex represented by Ea ΔG, ΔH and ΔS were determined.

INTRODUCTION

The thermodynamic and kinetic parameters associated with the binding of secreted mouse prolactin to mouse hepatic recptors were investigated. When the reaction temperature was incrased from 8 to 37c the association rate constant K+1, increased approximately 5 fold (240).

The thermodynamic for the reversible denaturation of chemotrypsinogen have been studied by the difference spetrum technique (283), the results are analyzed to provide continous value of the standard free energy, enthalpy and intropy terms over the temperature range from 0 to 65c and over the pH range from 0,5 to 3.7.

In order to gain deeper insight to the molecular basis of ^{99m}Tc-MDP-HSA or bone complexes, the kinetic and thermodynamic parameters governing the complexes formation of ^{99m}Tc-MDP to these proteins were carried out through investigation of the effect of time (time-course) and temperature on the equilibrium binding constants, the value of association and dissociation rate constans were determined.

5.1 THE KINETIC STUDIES

5.1.1 the time-course of ^{99m}Tc-MDP binding to its binding protein (HAS):

1- at zero time 100µl of ^{99m}Tc-MDP (2.8x10^{-6}M), were incubated with 100µl of HSA (1mg/,1) the final volume was

500μl made up by adding phosphate buffer pH 7.4, the reaction mixture was incubated at 37c for several time intervals (20, 30, 45, & 60min).

2- after each time interval, the assay tubes were with drawn and then applied to the surface of sephadex-G100 gel-filteration column (1.5x30cm) equilibrated with phosphate buffer pH 7.4. elution was carried out using the same buffer to separate bound ^{99m}Tc-MDP-HSA complex from free ^{99m}Tc-MDP, the flow rate was 12ml/h and fraction volume of 2ml.

3- radioactivity of each fraction tube in cpm was measured using gamma counter.

4- parallel experiments were performed to determine the amount of non-specific binding.

5- to determine the time-course of the association of ^{99m}Tc-MDP with its binding protein at different temperatures, the above experiment was performed at further three temperatures (20, 30 and 50°c).

Calculation:

1- the value of ^{99m}Tc-MDP bound specifically in picomole ^{99m}Tc-MDP per mg protein was calculated according to the following formula:

2- the values of specific binding (SB) of ^{99m}Tc-MDP (pmol/mg protein) were plotted against the time of incubation.

5.1.2 the time –course of ^{99m}Tc-MDP binding to BBP bone homogenate:-

1- at zero time, 100μl of bone homogenate (BBP) was incubated with 100μl ^{99m}Tc-MDP (2.8×10^{-6}M), the final volume was completed to 500μl with phosphate buffer pH 7.4 the reaction mixture was incubated at 37c for several time intervals (15, 30, 45, and 60 min).

2- after each time interval, the reaction tubes were with drawn and applied to the surface of sephadex-G100 column (1.0x30cm) equilibrated with phosphate buffer pH 7.4, elution was carred out with same buffer above.

3- steps (3-5) of experiment 5.1.1 were followed and repeated to each interval.

Calculation:

1- the percentage of the specific binding of ^{99m}Tc-MDP in (M) were determined as in experiment 5.1.1.

2- the values of SB% were plotted vs time intervals.

5.1.3 determination of hill coefficient (n) of ^{99m}Tc-MDP binding to its binding sites of HSA:

1- 100μl of HSA was incubated with 100μl ^{99m}Tc-MDP at 37c for 30 minutes, the final volume was completed to 500μl using phosphate buffer pH 7.4.

2- the steps 2-4 of experiment 5.1.1 were carried out as mentioned before.

Calculation:

1- the values of ^{99m}Tc-MDP bound specifically (M) were calculated as in experiment 5.1.1.

2- the hill-coefficient were obtained using the following equation (hill equation):

n log L= log Kd + log (Bspecific)/(Bmax-Bspecific)

where L=free ^{99m}Tc-MDP concentration in the incubation medium.

3- log (Bspecific) / (Bmax-Bspecific) was ploted against log L, the stope the straight line give the hill coefficient (n) value.

5.1.4 determination of the hill coefficient ^{99m}Tc-MDP binding to bone homogenate (BBP):

1- 100µl of BBP was incubated with 100µl ^{99m}Tc-MDP at 37c for 30 minutes, the final volume 500µl was made up by adding phosphate buffer pH 7.4.

2- the steps 2-4 of experiment 5.1.1 were repeated as mentioned before.

Calculation:

The same calculation used as in experiment 5.1.3.

5.2 THE THERMODYNAMIC STUDIES

5.2.1 the thermodynamic of the ^{99m}Tc-MDP binding to HSA:

The same steps mentioned in experiment (5.1.3) were followed exactly and the expeniment was carried out at four temperatures (20, 30, 37 and 50°c).

Calculation:

1- the thermodynamic parameters of standard state were obtained from van't hoff equation, the values of the natural log of equilibrium constants (affinity constants Ka) abtained at different temperatures were plotted vs the reciprocal values of absolute temperature in Kelvin (1/T) according to the following equation:

In Ka= $(\Delta S/R) - (\Delta H/RT)$

Were ΔH = the enthalpy change of the standard state. ΔS=the enthalpy change of the standard state. R= the gas constant that equals to 8.341 J/K, ΔH value obtained from the slope of the straight line of the diagram. The change in Gibbs free energy of the standard state ΔG was obtained from the following equation:

ΔG= RT ln Ka

While the standard state entropy change was obtained from

$\Delta S = (\Delta H - \Delta G) / T$

2- the thermodynamic parameters of transition state were obtained from Arrhenius plot of in K+1 or Bmax (in biochemical reactions) (287) values against 1/T gives alinear relationship according to the following equation:

In K+1 (or Bmax = in A-(Ea/RT)

Where A = Arrhenius constant or frequency factor. The value of apparent energy of activation (Ea) of the binding reaction can be determined from the slope of the straigt line. The enthalpy of transition state (ΔH^*) can be obtained from:

$\Delta H^* = Ea - RT$

Transition state free energy change is found by using the following equation:

$\Delta G^* = RT$ IN K+1 + RT in (KT/h)

(K, h) are Boltzmann and planks constants respectively. The change in entropy of the transition state ΔS^* is found from the following relation :

$\Delta S^* = (\Delta H^* - \Delta G^*)/T$

5.2.2 the thermodynamic of the ^{99m}Tc-MDP binding to BBP:

The same step mentioned in experiment 5.1.4 were followed exactly and the experiment was performed at four temperatures (20, 30, 37 and 50°c)

Calculation :

As explained in the experiment (5.2.1)

RESULTS AND DISCUSSION

1- kinetic of the ^{99m}Tc-MDP binding to HSA and BBP:

The time course of the binding of ^{99m}Tc-MDP to HSA:

The time course of the formation of ^{99m}Tc-MDP-HSA complex at four different temperature (20, 30, 37 and 50°c) were shown in fig (5.1). the concentration of complex formed ^{99m}Tc-MDP-HSA after time (t) was calculated from the following equation:

$$\left[^{99m}Tc\text{-}MDP\text{-}HSA\right] = \frac{counts(cpm\ )of\ ^{99m}Tc\text{-}MDP\ specificaly\ bound\ after\ time(\ t\ )}{Total\ count(\ cpm\ )\ of\ ^{99m}Tc\text{-}MDP\ used\ in\ the\ incubation\ tube} \times conc\ of\ ^{99m}Tc\text{-}MDP\ in(\ M\ )used$$

in molar formed after time(t)

The results of time –course programmes at different temperatures revealed that the binding of ^{99m}Tc-MDP to its binding albumin is a temperature and time dependant with maximum binding occurs at 37c and equilibrium took place after 30 min of reaction time, while there is no equi;ibrium at 50c, there is arapid decrease happened after 30 min this is may be due to the denaturation of protein in this temperature, or may be due to the change in the oxidation state of ^{99m}Tc and this caused areverse reaction and dissociasion of the complex formed. Increasing the temperature from 20c to 37c the bound ^{99m}Tc-MDP to albumin was incrased 12.9% while incrased 10.44% when the reaction temperature increased from 30c to 37°c.

The time-course of association of ^{99m}Tc-MDP with its binding site in BBP:

162

Fig (5.2) represent the time-course for the formation of complex of ^{99m}Tc-MDP with BBP at four different temperatre (20, 0, 37 and 50°c). the maximum binding was occurred after 30-45 minutes. Increasing the temperature from 20c to 30, 37 and 50°c the specifically bound of ^{99m}Tc-MDP to bone homogenate were increased 13.06%, 20.48% and 2.74% respectively, these results indicate that the binding of ^{99m}Tc-MDP to bone homogenate is temperature dependant. Luis and frank indicate that the inding of 125I-iodosmPRL (secreted mouse prolactin) o mouse hepatic receptors reached equilibrium after 4000 sec. of incubation time at 37°c (240). Hubbard and klee indicate that the binding of 125I-CaM to CaM-dependant phosphaase reached equilibrium after 48 min. of incubation using 200ng of phosphatase and only 100 fold of ^{125}I-CaM would be bound (284).

Agree etal. Showed that the time-course of Ca_{+2}-dependentbinding of ^{125}I-CaM to erythrocyte membrane reached equilibrium after 240 minutes giving 4 pmole ^{125}I-CaM bound/mg membrane proteins (285).

Determination of kineic parameters of ^{99m}Tc-MDP binding to HSA :

The time – course of ^{99m}Tc-MDP binding to its binding HSA was carried out to describe the kinetic parameters of the binding. The simplest proposed model represnting the interaction of ^{99m}Tc-MDP with albumin could be expresd by the following:

^{99m}Tc-MDP + HSA → ^{99m}Tc-MDP-HSA

K+1 is the rate of the association of ^{99m}Tc-MDP with its binding site in HSA, and K represents the rate of the reverse reaction i.e, the dissociation of the complex formed under the same conditions.

$$ka = \frac{\left[^{99m}Tc-MDP-HSA\right]}{\left[^{99m}Tc-MDP\right]\left[HSA\right]} \quad \& \quad k_d = \frac{\left[^{99m}Tc-MDP\right]\left[HSA\right]}{\left[^{99m}Tc-MDP-HSA\right]} \text{ At equilibrium}$$

$$\text{Thus } Ka = 1/K_d = K_{+1}/K_1$$

Where Ka is the equilibrium constant of the association and Kd is the equilibrium constant of dissociation of the complex. The value of Ka and total concentration of protein binding sites (Bmax) were cacuated from sctchard plot at four different temperatures.

Time- course data shown in fig (5.1) fit the second order kinetics for the association of ^{99m}Tc-MDP with its binding sites in HSA as illustrated in the following equation (286):

$$K_{+1} = \frac{1}{t} \times \frac{\bar{X}}{\bar{X}^2 - R_o L_o} \left(\ln \frac{\bar{X} - X}{R_o L_o - \bar{X}x} + \ln \frac{R_o L_o}{\bar{X}} \right)$$

Where K+1 is the kinetic association constant inM-1 S-1, L0 is the total ^{99m}Tc-MDP concentration in molar, R0, the total concentration of the HSA – binding sites (Bmax),

X the concentration of ^{99m}Tc-MDP-HSA complex formed at equilibrium, and X, is the concentration of the complex formed after time (t) (286). When ln (X-X/ (R0L0-XX) is plotted as aunction of time (t), alinear plot shown in most cases ascertained that the reaction fit second order kinetic and conforms to the rate law of equation (2) K+1 can be calculated from the slope of the lot. The values for the dissociation rate constant K-1 were also determined from the formula (287):

$$K-1 = K+1 (R \ L \ / \ X)........(3)$$

Where L is the concentration of free ^{99m}Tc-MDP at equilibrium and equal to (L0-X), and the concentration of free binding site at equilibrium R is equal to (R-X). the Ka values were also obtained from equation (1). Fig (5.3) and (5.4) represent the kinetics of complex formation between ^{99m}Tc-MDP and HSA at different temperatures (20, 30, 37°c) the results indicated that the association rate constant K+1 decreased with ncreasing temperature. On increasing temperature from 20c to 37c K+1 decreased by 45% the dissociaton rate constant K1 of the complex formed between ^{99m}Tc-MDP and HSA was increased with increasing temperature. On increasing the reaction temperature from 20°c to 37°c K-1 increased by 13.7% this means that the complex formed is more stable at low temperature.

The results obtained from table (5.1) indicate that the affinity of ^{99m}Tc-MDPto form stable complex with HSA is very high, but it was decreased with increasing temperature, this phonomena may be due to the change in the suitable conformation of the protein and affect the suitable binding sites.

Determination of the kinetic parameters of ^{99m}Tc-MDP bndin to BBP:

Fig (5.4) represent the kinetics of complex formation between ^{99m}Tc-MDP and BBP of bone homogenate at different temperatures. The time-course data and equilibrium for the binding of ^{99m}Tc-MDP to its binding sites in BBP of bone homogenate he same mathematical formula and reactions were used and applied to determine the reaction kinetics. He time-course data of binding followed the second order kinrtic, table (5.2) show the association constant K+1 and dissociation constant at (20, 30 and 37°c), the resultes show that K+1 increased with increasing the reaction temperature, K+1 was increased by 11.3% when the temperature was increased from 20 to 37c while K1 was decreased by 105% when the reaction emperaure was increased from 30 to 37c these results indicate that the ^{99m}Tc-MDP have a high stability to form a complex with bone containing protein, or to the bone homogenate (BBP).

Ka values which were calculated from K+1 and K1 table (5.2) show very high affinity of ^{99m}Tc-MDP to form stable complex with BBP of bone homogenate. But in general the Ka or Kd values were less than the corespounding value with ^{99m}Tc-MDP-HSA, this phenomena may be due to the low protein or gamma-

166

carboxyglutaic acid protein in bone matrix hence low binding sites, and then low Bmax value were observed in case of bone homogenate than that with HSA at that temperature. Bmax in case of ^{99m}Tc-MDP-HSA at 37°c was more than that of BBP of bone bonogeneate by 119.3% at the same temperature. Hooper and Kelly studied the binding of cholinergic synapic vesicales in rat brain, they found that the Kd and Bmax value were 10nm and 80pmol/mg respectively and the binding reaction followed a second order kinetic with association rate equal to 3.1x106m-1s, dissociation rate of 1.3x10-2s-1. (18).

Determination of hill coefficient (n) of ^{99m}Tc-MDP binding to HSA and BBP of bone homogenate:

When hill equation (260), was applied to the results obtained from scatchard analysis, the cooperativiy of the bindingsites of ^{99m}Tc-MDP can be evaluated through the determination of hill coefficient (n). fig (5.5) represent the hill plot of ^{99m}Tc-MDP binding to HSA, the results sow that hill coefficient for this binding was 1.7, this value indicate that the reaction between ^{99m}Tc-MDP and HSA is characterized by high affinity and cooperativity. Many authors have reported that when the hill coefficient was ranged between (1-2) this indicate that reaction have a high affinity and cooperativity (244, 288-290).

Fig (5.6) show the hill plot of the binding of ^{99m}Tc-MDP to BBP of bone homogenate, the plot show a linear relationship with

167

slope of 1.16. this value indicate that a cooperative interactions may be present (291).

The thrmodynamics of the binding of ^{99m}Tc-MDP to its binding sites in HSA and of bone homogenate:

(A) thermodynamic parameters at standard state:

Fig (5.7) represent the dependence of the equilibrium binding constant for the binding of ^{99m}Tc-MDP to HSA and BBP of bne homogenate on the temperature (van't hoff plot). The ΔH values were calculated from the slope of the curves. Table (5.5) and (5.6) indicate that the reaction of HSA with ^{99m}Tc-MDP is slightly exothermic (with negative ΔH value), while ΔH has a positive value in case of BBP of bone homogenate, table (5.6), i.e. the reaction of ^{99m}Tc-MDP with BBP of bone homogenate is slightly endothermic reaction. ΔG values were negative in case of HSA and BBP of bone homogenate his reflects the stability of the complex hence the high affinity of the reactions.

The negative values of ΔG for the binding reactions are controlled by positively ΔS value , so this means that the reaction of ^{99m}Tc-MDP with both HSA and BBP of bon homogenate are characterized by the sole contribution of ΔS to the stability of the complexes formed while ΔH has little or no effect. The small positive value of ΔH in case of bone homogenate may indicate afavorable interaction between groups within both ^{99m}Tc-MDP and BBP or bone hydroxyapatite. These include the non covalent interactions which are fundamentally electrostatic in nature such as charge – charge interactions which occur in both MDP and its binding materal in bone homogenate, other type of interaction include charge-dipole, dipole-dipole, charge-induced dipole, dipole-induced dipole and hydrogen bond. The sum of these types of interactions can yield some stabilization to the folded structure of the complex in case of protein binding with MDP. So the negative value of ΔG showed that the overall reaction was energetically favorable in the dirction of complex formation. The positive entropy change was the major force driving this reaction and indicate that hydrophobic interactions play an important role in stabilizing the complex formation (292).

The negative value of ΔG and positive values of ΔS in ^{99m}Tc-MDP – HSA reaction are nearly identical with its values for ^{99m}Tc-MDP – bone complex at four different temperature indicate that the ^{99m}Tc-MDP has a good affinity to bind HSA and bone matrix, and the complex formed is stable at these conditions.

B- the thermodynamic parameters of transition state:

According to the transition state theory, the interaction of two proteis lead to the formation of an activated complx (transition state), then the formation of the final product.

^{99m}Tc-MDP + ligand $\rightarrow$ (^{99m}Tc-MDP-ligand) $\rightarrow$ ^{99m}Tc-MDP-lig-complex

Initial state   transition state   final state

On application of Arrhenius equation to the kineic data. The transition state thermodynamic parameters could be determined. Fig (5.8.A and B) show that the dependence of maximum binding capacity (Bmax) for the binding of ^{99m}Tc-MDP to HSA and BBP of bone homogenate on temperature (Arrhenius plot). The results obtained were show in tale 5.3 and 5.4, the high positive values of ΔG^* indicate that the formation of an activated complex was non spontaneous process and require a lot of energy eqal to (Ea) to overcome the transition state energy barrier and giving the final product, whereas negative ΔS^* value revealed that the activated complex had more order structure than the reactants.

The ctivation energy (Ea) required o overcome the transition stae enrgy barrier in case of ^{99m}Tc-MDP reaction with HSA is more than Ea required in case of ^{99m}Tc-MDP-bone complex. The results indicate that the formation of complex with bone is more easier than that of HSA cases bone and albumin complexation with MDP, the activated ------ MDP-complex possessed a more oder than the reactants ---- (AS*<0). Table 5.5 and 5.6 shows that the thermodynamic parameters of the standard state and transition state of the reaction of ^{99m}Tc-MDP with HSA and BBP of bone homogenate the results of both tabes may----- the following equations:

(1) ΔH value for ^{99m}Tc-MDP – binding with HSA is exothermic s---- while that of ^{99m}Tc-MDP with BBP of bone homogenate was ---- endothermic.

(2) ΔG values for both reactions ae negative, it is slightly negative in case of HSA by 4.9 KJ at (37˚c) than that of BBP of bone homogenate.

(3) ΔS values for the reaction of ^{99m}Tc-MDP with HSA and BBP of bone homogenate are nearly have the same positive values.

(4) the activation energy Ea required for the formation of transition complex with HSA is more than that with BBP of bone homogenate by about 2KJ mol, and there is small increase in ΔH* in the reaction of MDP with HSA than with BBP of bone homogenate at the same temperature.

Determination of binding – reaction according to the thermodynamics parameters using equilibrium data give an overall idea about the nature of forces controlling the complex formation. Comparasion of the values of \ H* ΔG* and ΔS* of transition state with those of standard state in table 5.5 and 5.6, lead to choose a thermodynamic model (293). Our model proposes the existence of three thermodynamic states fig (5.9), state (A) represent the intital energy level of the isolated hydrated species. State (B) the components have come together and mutually penetrated their hydration sphere to form a partially immobilized hydrophobically associated species. State (C) represent the fully interacting ^{99m}Tc-MDP-complex. In step

(1) the binding of ^{99m}Tc-MDP was associated with positive ΔG^* value, this indicate that the initial step of the reaction requires input of energy for the system.

The negative entropy change (ΔS^*) for step of the reaction reflects the change of ^{99m}Tc-MDP – complex (transition complex) to a more ordered structure. The positive value of ΔH^* shows that the heat content of the activated complex is more than of isolated species. Partial immobilization of the hydrophobically associated complex formed, in step 1, occurs when isolated hydrated species i.e. ^{99m}Tc-MDP and HSA or BBP interact partially so that there is a mutual penetration of their hydration layers to form the activated complex. The hydrophilic amino acid residues which were previously accessible to solvent in the isolated-subunits become buried upon complex formation and hence produce an increase in the number of released water molecules, thus, the negative value of ΔS^* is due to the loss of a number of translational and rotational deress of freedom originally present in both isolated species or the water molecules that have been ordered will then be released and gain freedom of motion.

In the second step of protein association the hydrophobically associated species (state B) participaes in further interactions as illusterated in state C, giving the fully-interacting association species. So step 2 is a description of intermolecular interactions betwwn ^{99m}Tc-MDP and its binding proteins. The formation of protein-protein or proein-

REFERENCE

1. Manuel T., and walterw., (1976), rediopharmacy, awitly-interscoence publication. Chapter 1.

2. Hine G.J., Sorenson j, a, (1974), instrumentation in nuclear medicine, vol.1, 2, new york. Academic press.

3. Colombetti L.G, (1979), principles of rediopharmacy, vol.1-3, boca raton florida. CRC press.

4. Stang L.G, Jr, radionuclide generator, (1969), BNL report no, 13595, CONF690413-1, U.S.A tomic energy commission, Oak ridge.

5. Myers W.G, (1966), radioactive pharmaceuticals, usa atomic energy commission, oak ridge, p.217.

6. Lederer C.M, Hollander J.m, and perlman l., (1967), table of isotopes 6 th ed wiley, new york.

7. Obrien H.A, and ogard A, (1973), J. nucl. Med., 14, 635.

8. Welch M.J., lifton J.f, and ter-pogossian M.M., (1969), J. label comp. radiopharm, 5, 168.

9. Gelbard A.S., hara T., tilbury R.S., and langhlin J.S., (1973) radiopharmacuticals and labeled compound, JAEA vienna, p.239.

10. Ratusky J., and tykva R., (1967) J. label comp, radiopharm. 3, 50.

11. Vercier P, and bidault J.P., (1968), bull, soc. Chim. Fr. 3915.

12. Vervier P., (1981). J. label comp. radiopharm., 4.19.

13. Bayly R.J., (1966). Nucleonics, 24 (6), 46.

14. Collipp P.J., Kaplan S.A., boyle D.C, shimizi C.S.N., and ling S.M., (1965), nature (London), 207, 876.

15. Taylor R.T., and weissbach h., (1971), J. boil. Chem., 242, 1517.

16. Turner J.C., (1967), J. label. Comp. radiopharm, 3, 217.

17. Putman E.W, and hassid w.z., (1972), J. boil. Chem.., 196-749.

18. Walton G.N., (1964), radiochim. Acta., 108.

19. Lifton J. F., and Welch M.J., (1971), radiat. Res., 45, 35.

20. Wolfgang R., (1965), ann. Rev. phys. Chem.., 16, 15.

21. Svoboda K, (1987), radiochemical acta, 41, 83.

22. Gelbard A.S., tilbury R.S, and Laughlin J.S., (1989), radiopharmaceutical and labeled compounds, IAE A., Vienna.

23. Albert f.C., and Geoffrey W., (1972), advanced inorganic chemistry, 2nd ed, wiley eastern o. l., (960).

24. Baolar J. C., emeleus H. J., ranald n., and toroman A.f., (1973), comprehensive inorganic chemistry vol. (3), pergamon press, new york.

25. Deutch E., libson k., jurisson S., and lndoy L.F., (1983) progress in inorganic chemistry vol. (30), 75.

26. Fiser M., brabec V., dragoun o., laznickova A., kovalic a, and rysavy m, (1986), int. J. ppl. Radiat. Isot., 73, 1213.

27. Davison A., and jones A.g, (1982), int. J. appl. Radiat. Isot., 33, 875.

28. Jones A.G., and Davison A, (1982). Int. J. appl. Radiat. Isot., 33, 867.

29. Thomas C., Carla P.D, Daniel J.h., martin V.M., and george M. W., (1985), J. of chem.. edu., 62 (11), 965.

30. Tji T. G., vink H.A., gelsema w.J., & deligny C.L., (1990) int. J. appl. Radiat. Isot., 41 (1), 17.

31. Abdel –dayem H.M., (1989), second seicientific conference of Iraqi atomic energy commission , November, p.294.

32. Thieme K., (1988), int.J. appl. Radiat. Isot., 39 (3). 267.

33. Kennedy C.M.. mikelsons M.V., Lawson B.L. & pinkerton i.C. , (1988), int.J. appl.radiat. isot, 39 (3), 213.

34. Moore P.W., shying M.E., sodeau J.M., evans J.V., maddalena D.J., and farrington k.h., (1987), int.J. appl. Redial. Isot., 38 (1), 25.

35. Kokta L., hospes M., vlcek J., & husak V., (1978), radiochem radioanal. Lett., 33 (3), 149.

36. Guyton A. C., (1971), medical physiology, 4th ed, w.B. saunders philadelephia, chap.20.

37. Kemmitt R. D., and oeacock R.D., (1973), the chemistry of manganese, technetium and rehenium, pergamon press.

38. Eckelman W.C., and levenson S.M., (1977), int j appl. Radiat isotopes, 28, 67.

39. Schwochau K., (1978), angew, chem., 102, 329.

40. Libson K., deutsch E., and Barnett B.L., (1980), J.am. chem.. soc., 102, 2476.

41. Steigman J., meinken G., and Richards O., (1975), int. J. appl. Radiat. Isot., 26, 601.

42. Munze R., (1980), radiocchem, radioanal, lett., 43, 219.

43. Russell C.D., & cash A.g, (1979), J.nucl. med., 20, 532.

44. Loberg M.D., coder E.h., fields A.T., and callery P.S., (1979), J. nucl. Med., 20, 1181.

45. Johannsen, B., berger, R., and schomacker k., (1980). Radiochem radional lett, 42, 177.

46. Johannsen, B., training course lecture (1986), report J.G., 26/60/85.

47. Peter J.E., and Edward S.w., (1981), nuclear medicine. An interoducation text, black well sciantifc publication chapter (1).

48. Gal E., grenier R.p., Schmidt D.h., & port S.C., (1990), eur.J. nuel med., 16 (1), 11.

49. Blauenstein p.A., (1986), swiss pharma, 8 (Ab), 24.

50. Fogelman, I., hay I.D., citrin D.l., (1980), brt. J. radiol, 53, 874.

51. Chauhan Y.P.S., chander J., and pyshpa M., (1990), nucl. Med. Boil., 17 (4), 401.

52. Baum R.P., happ J., maul F.D, standke R., & hor G., (1985), nukl. Mediz., 24 (3), 141.

53. Kung H.F. molnar M., billings J., and wicks R., (1984), J. nucl. Med., 25, 326.

54. Moretti J.L., defer G., cinotti L. casaro o., degos J.D., et al, (1990), eur J. nucl. Med., 16 (1), 17.

55. Juri P.N., linder k., feld T., trcher E.N., & nunn A.D., (1988), nuki mediz, 24, 711.

56. Narra R.k., nunn A.D., kuezynski B.L., feld t, wedeking P., & eckelmen W.C., (1989), J.nucl. med., 30, 1830.

57. Narra R.k., numm A.D., kuczynski B.l., dirocco R.J., feld T., silva A. D., & eckelman W.C., (1990), J.nucl. med., 31, 1370.

58. Zmbova B., & konstantinouska-djokc D., (1987), isotopen praxis, 23, 278.

59. Weiner I.M., and mudgw G.h., (1964), am J. med., 36, 743.

60. Toothaker A.k., adelstein S.J., & kassis A.I., (1984), J. nucl. Med. Boil., 11, 225.

61. Raynaud C., (1979), principles of radiopharmacology, CRC press, pocaration, vol. (3), page 89.

62. Kagi J. H.R., himmelhoch S.R., whagner P.D., (1974), J.biol. chem.., 249, 3537.

63. Davison A., sohn M., and orvig C., (1980), J. nucl, med., 20, 168.

64. Cheruv l.R., numm A.D., and loberg M.D., (1982), sem. Nucl. Med., 12, 5.

65. Meyer-brunot H.G., and kuberl H., (1968), am. J. physiol, 214, 1193.

66. Burns h.D., marzilli l.G., sowa D., vaum D., and wagner H.N., (1977), J. nucl. Med., 18, 624.

67. Kato-azuma M., (1982), int. J. appl. Radiat. Isot., 33, 937.

68. Nunn A.D., and loberg M.d, (1981), in radiopharamaceuticals, structure activity relationships, (spencer R.P., editor), grune & Stratton new yorj, chap, 25.

69. Deutch E., glavan, sod V.J., (1981), J. nucl. Med., 22, 897.

70. Deutch E., bushong W., glavan K.A., (1981), seience, 214, 84.

71. Nishiyama H., deutsch E., and Adolph R., (1982), J. nucl, med., 23, 1093.

72. Deutsch E., libson k., and vanderheyden, J., (1982), J. nucl. Med., 23, 9.

73. Vanderheyden J., libson K., and nosco D., (1983), int. J. appl. Radiat. Isot., 34, 1611.

74. Thakurm M. , and park C., (1984), int, J. appl. Radiat. Isot., 35, 507.

75. Schwochau k., lines k.H., steinmetz h.J., and astheimer l., (1993), nucl. Med. Boil., 20 (3), 317.

76. Holman B.l., jones A.G., jemes J.l., and Davison A., (1984), J. nucl. Med., 25, 1350.

77. Willerson J., parkry R., and lewis S., J. cardiovasc. Med., (1982), 3, 291.

78. Bianco J., kemper A., and taylor A., (1983), J. nucl. Med., 24, 485.

79. Bevan J., tofe A., benedict J., francis, and Barnett B., (1980), J. nucl. Med., 21, 967.

80. Al-Janabi M. A., and Abdul-Hussein M. kadim, (1983), int. J. appl. Radiat. Isot., 34, 1473.

81. Treher E.N., francessconi L.C., gougoutas J.Z., malley M.F., & nunn A.D., (1989), inorg. Chem.., 28, 3411.

82. Genant H. K., bautovich G.h., and singh M., (1974), radiology, 113, 373.

83. Cohn S.R., lippinott S.w, and gusmano E.A., (1963), radiat. Res., 19-104.

84. Wilson J.S., genant h.k, and hattner R.S., (1978), radiology, 126, 185.

85. Hikaru S., fumishige I., ryusuke f., tetsuyak., masao k., and makoto n., (1993), nucl. Med. Boil. , 20 (3), 337.

86. Subramanian G., and mcafee J.G, (1971), radiology, 99, 192.

87. Sy W.M., (1974), J. nucl. Med., 15, 1089.

88. Huigen y.M., krips h.j, hullemans, gelsema W.J., & deligny C.l., (1990), int. J. appl. Radiat. Isot., 41, 189.

89. Subramanian G., mcafee J.G., blair R.T., omara R.R., and raston P.H., (1972), radiology, 102, 701.

90. Jobn R.B., domininc L., geert E., rolfde J., & peter J.E., (1990), eur. J. nucl. Med., 16 (8-10), 649.

91. Perez R., cohen Y., henry R., and panneciere C., (1972), J. nucl. Med., 13, 788.

92. Subramanian G., mcafee J.G., blair R.J., & kallfez F.A., (1975), J.nucl. med., 16, 744.

93. Castronovo jr.F.P., and Callahan R.J., (1972), J. nucl. Med., 13, 823.

94. Subramanian G., mcafee J.G., blair R.J., rosenstrich M., CoCo M., and Duxbury C.E., (1975), J. nucl. Med., 16, 1137.

95. Ackerhalt R.E., blau M., and bakshi S., (1974), J. nucl. Med., 15, 1153.

96. Weber D.A., keyes J.W., and Wilson JR.G.A., (1976), radiology, 120, 615.

97. Schavrz A., and kloss G., (1981), J. nucl. Med., 22, 77.

98. Buell U., kleinhans E., & zorn-bopp E., (1982), J.nucl.med. , 23, 214.

99. Dalrich B.U., carl-martin k., eduard k., & brigette J., (1983), J.nucl. med., 24 (12), 1201.

100. Raymakers J.A., savelkoul T.J., Hoekstra A., vidder W.J. etal., (1990), eur.J. nucl. Med., 16 (3), 157.

101. Brattsev V.A., danilova G.N., tarasov N.F., & koval chuk N.D., (1986), J. label. Comp. & radiopharm, XXIII, 1428.

102. Wang T.S.T., mojdehi G.E., fawwaz R.A. & Johnson p.M., (1979), J. nucl. Med., 20, 1066.

103. Wang T.S.T., fawwaz R.A., Johnson L.J., mojdehi G.E., and Johnson P.M., (1980), J.nucl.med., 21, 767.

104. Bevan J.A.: tofe A.J., benedict J.J., francis M.D., & Barnett B.l., (1980), J.nucl.med., 21, 961.

105. Tanabe S., zodda J.P., libsosk, deutsch, E., & heineman w.R., (1983), int.J. appl.radiat.isot., 34, 1585.

106. Schumichec C., Schmidt h., & koutsomains D., (1982), J. nucl. Med., 23, 77.

107. Domstad P.A., coupal J.J., kim E.E., blake J.S., and deland f.h., (1980), radiology, 136, 209.

108. Resenthall l., arzoumanian A., damtew B.U., & tremblay J., (1981), clin. Nucl. Med., 6, 353.

109. Fogelman I., (1980), eur, J. nucl. Med., 5,473.

110. Gropal S., & Thomas A., (1983), radiology, 149, 823.

111. Citrin D.l., bessent R.G., & greig w.R., (1977), clin.radiol., 28, 107.

112. Jones A.G., francis M.D., & davis M.A., (1976), seminar in nucl. Med., 6, 3.

113. Tofe A.J., & ftancis M.D., (1974), J. nucl. Med., 15, 69.

114. Wang T.S.T, hsain p., & spencer R.p., (1978), J.nucl. med., 19.1151.

115. Davis M.A., & jones A.g, (1976), sem. Nucl. Med., 6, 19.

116. Citrin D.L., bessent R.G., tuohyj B., elms T., mc ginlay E., greig W.R., & blumgart l.h., (1975), brit. J. radiol., 48, 118.

117. Bergquist L., strand S.E., hafstrom L., & jonsson P.E., (1984), eur. J. nucl. Med., 9, 129.

118. Forgelmam i., bessent R.G., tuner J.G., citrin D.L., boyle I.T., & greig W.R., (1978), J. nucl. Med., 19, 270.

119. Zimmer A.M., isitman A.T., & holmes R., (1975), J. nucl. Med., 16, 352.

120. Shani J., amir D., soskolne W.A., (1990), J.nucl. med., 31, 2011.

121. Deligny cl.l., gelsema W.J., tji T.G., huygen y.M., & vink H.A., (1990), nucl. Med. Boil., 17, 161.

122. Anderson P., vaugham A.T.M., & varley N.R., (1988), nucl. Med. Boil., 15, 293.

123. Hambbright P., mcrae J., valk P.E., bearden A.J., & Shipley B.A., (1975), J. nucl. Med., 16, 478.

124. Korteland J., dekker B.G., & lignyde C.l., (1980), int. J. appl. Radiate. Isot., 31, 315.

125. Claessens R.A., vander linden J.M., schimitz J.E., & jong de N.H., (1985), inorg. Chim. Acta., 109, 123.

126. Mulder G., Oldenburg S.J., van Oort W.J., & den hartigh J., (1981), int. J. appl. Radiat. Iso., 32, 675.

127. Russell C.D., & cash A.G., (1978), int. J. appl. Radiat. Isot., 30, 485.

128. Kalincak M., machan V., & vilcek S., (1981), int. J. appl. Radiat. Isot., 32, 493.

129. Vilcek S., machan V., kalincak M., (1984), int. J. appl. Radiate. Isot., 35, 228.

130. Vilcek S., kalincak M., machan V., (1985), J. radioanal. Nucl. Chem.., 88, 359.

131. Savelkoul T.J., Oldenburg S.J., van Oort W.J., & dursama S.A., (1984), int. J. appl. Radiat. Isot., 35, 709.

132. Mikelsons M.V., & pinkerton T.C., (1986), anal. Chem.., 58, 1007.

133. Deutsch E., libson k., becker C.B., francis M.D., tofe A.J., ferguson D.l., & mccreary L.D., (1980), J. nucl. Med., 21, 859.

134. Subramanian G., and mcafee J.G., (1973), J. nucl. Med., 14, 640.

135. Mele M., elio C., angelo f., domenico p., maria p., & amgelo d'addabbo, (1983), J. nucl. Med., 24, 334.

136. Pauwels E.K., blom J., camps J.A., herman J., & R.J. ke A.M., (1983) eur J. nucl. Med., 8, 118.

137. Rigo P., (1990), eur. J. nucl. Med., 16 (3), 179.

138. Tuomo lantto. (1999), eur. J. nucl. Med., 16. 677.

139. Gunilla M.G., laes A., soren M., & per-anders A., (1990), eur. J. nucl. Med., 16, 671.

140. Chervu L.R., nunn A.D., & loberg M.D., (1982), semin. Nucl. Med., 12, 5.

141. Wynchank S., mann M.D., & gonin R., (1990), eur. J. nucl. Med., 16 , 337.

142. Steen L.N., bente p., eiliv S., & lnge R., (1990), eur. J. nucl. Med., 16 (8-10). 639.

143. Henderson M.J., wastin M.l. , brominge M., Selwyn P., & smith A., (1990), clin. Radiol. , 41, 411.

144. Fogelman I., (1982), eur. J. nucl., med., 7, 506.

145. Fogelman I., & bessent R.G., (1980), J. nucl. Med., 21, 296.

146. Seto H., futatsuya R. & ihara F, (1984), radiat. Med., 2, 87.

147. Al-jnabi M.A., moussa S.O., (1990), J. labell. Comp. & radiopharm, XXIII (5), 519.

148. Molinoff P.B., wolfe B.B., & weilland, (1981), life sci, 29, 427.

149. El-kolaly M.T., & el-wetery A.S., (1990), J. labell comp. & radiopharm, XXVIII (3), 329.

150. Lo J.M., piliai M.R., john C.S., & troutner D.E., (1990), int.J. appl. Radiat. Isot., 41 (1), 63.

151. Todorov B., nicolova M., eranz J., & svoboda i., (1989), 2nd scientific conference of IAEC, November, 274.

152. Vandef.E., stumpf E., bogl w., (1985), nuki. Mediz., 24 (2), 82.

153. Schumichen C., korfgen T., & Hoffmann G., (1980), nucl. Med., 19, 7.

154. Suha G.B., & boyd C.M., (1979), J. nucl. Med. Bed. Boil., 6, 201.

155. Huigen y.M., gelsema W.J., & de ligny C.l., (1990), int.J. appl. Radiat. Isot., 41 (3), 335.

156. Savelkoul T.J., van ginkel T.J., grouls R.J., oldenburgs. J., & duursma S.A., (1985), J. nucl. Med. Boil., 12, 125.

157. Grouls R.J., Oldenburg S.J., savelkoul T.J., & droge J.h., (1988), J. nucl. Med. Boil., 24, 127.

158. Vanlic R.N., joksmovic J., ristic B., tonic M., beatove S., & ajdinovic B., (1993), J. nucl. Med. Boil., 20 (3), 363.

159. Huggen y.M., tji T.G., gelsema W,J., de ligny C.l., (1989), int. J. appl. Radiat. Isot., 40, 629.

160. Salako Q., & theobald A.E., (1989), int. J. appl. Radiat. Isot., 40, 621.

161. Domenech R.G., Mendez O.A., alvarez J.G., marti, A.f., (1989), int. J. appl. Radiat. Isot., 40, 536.

162. Nakamura k., tukatani Y., kubo A., hashimoto S., (1989), eur. J. nucl. Med., 15, 100.

163. Streule k., de schrijver M., fridich R., (1988), nucl. Med. Comm.., 0, 59.

164. Corlija M., vokert W.A., john C.S., pillai M.R., lo J.M., troutner D.E., & holmes R.A., (1991) J. nucl. Med. Boil., 18, 167.

165. Block D., ogtrop M.V., arndt J.w., camps J.A., feittsma R.I., (1990), eur. J. nucl. Med., 16, 303.

166. Kroonenburgh M.JP., pauwels E.K.J.. (1988), nucl. Med. Comm.., 9,919.

167. Vanlic- razumenic N., petrovic J., & gorkic D., (1982), J. labell comp. & radiopharm, 19, 1568.

168. Vanlic-razumenic n., petrovic J., & gorkic D., (1984), eur. J. nucl. Med., 9, 370.

169. Richard S.T., georgeanna J.k, William C.k., William E.h., & Donald S.S., (1983), J. nucl. Med., 24, 224.

170. Kroesbergen J., gelsema W.J., & deligny C.l., (1985), J. nucl. Med. Boil., 12, 83.

171. Owunwanne A., o'mara R.E., & o'brien C., (1980), J. of radioanal. Chem.., 59 (2), 571.

172. Satz F.L., & thorne D.A., (1987), J. nucl. Med., 28, 820.

173. Mc carthy k., velchik M.G., alavia., mandell GA, esterhai J.l., & goll S., (1988), J. nucl. Med., 29, 1015.

174. Kodina G.E., (1986), J. label. Comp. & radiopharm. XXIII (10-12), 1432.

175. Richared P.S., (1990), nucl. Med. Boil., 17 (1), 73.

176. Littefield J.l., and rudd T.g, (1983), J. nucl. Med., 24 (6), 463.

177. Granowzka M., shepherd J., britton K.E., ward B., & mather, (1984), nucl. Med. Commun., 5, 485.

178. Locher J. th., Seybold k., anders R.Y., schubiger P.A., & march J.P., (1986), nucl. Med. Commun. , 7, 659.

179. Fritzberg A.R., (1987), nukl mediz, 26 (1), 7.

180. Eckelman W.C., paik C.H., & steigman J., (1989), nucl. Med. Boil., 16 (2) 171.

181. Saptogino A., becker W., wolf f., (1990), nukl. Mediz., 2, 54.

182. Duggleby R.G., (1981), anal. Biochem., 110, 9.

183. Rhodes B.A., zamoa P.O., newell k.D., & valdez E.F., (1986), J. nucl.med., 27, 685.

184. Lanterigne D., hnatwich D.J., (1984), int. J. appl. Radiat. Isot., 35, 617.

185. Maritta P., pirkko V., marja S., juhani H., & raijo V., (1990), eur. J. nucl. Med., 16, 621.

186. Yokoyama A., hata N., horiuchi k., masuda H., saji H., ohta H., & hamamoto K.,

187. Tamemasa O, goto R., takeda A., & Yano M., (1984), Radio isotopes, 33, 636.

188. Takeda A., goto R., & okada S., (1988), ann nucl. Med., 2, 55.

189. Atsushi T, & shoji O., (1989), int.J.appl.radiat.isot, 40 (7), 565.

190. Peter C.A., Elizabeth A.H., & Alistair M.S., (1977), plasma proteins analytical and preparative trchniques, Blackwell scientific publications. Oxford.pp.(160).

191. Levines, (1954), arch.biochem.biophys, 50, 515.

192. Mckernan W.M., & riketts C.R., (1960), biochem.J., 76, 117.

193. Kaldor G., saifer A,, & vecsler F., (1961), arch.biochem.biophys., 94, 207.

194. Gambal D., (1971), biochem.biophys.acta., 251, 54.

195. Shrivastava P.K, goch H., & zakrzewski k., (1972), biochim.biophys. acta, 271, 310.

196. Wichman A., & Anderson L.O, (1974), biochem, biophys. Acta., 372, 218.

197. Cohn E.j, strong l.e, Hughes w.l, mulford D.J., ashworth J.n., melin M., & taylor h.l, (1946). J.am. chem.. soc., 72, 454.

198. Herskovits T.T., & laskowski M., (1960), J. boil.chem., 235, pc 56.

199. Theodore T.H., & micheal L., (1962), J. boil. Chem.., 237, 2481.

200. Herskovits T.T, & laskowiski M., (1962) , J. boil. Chem.., 237, 3418.

201. Herskovits T.T, & mescantl L., (1965), J. bio. Chem.., 240, 639.

202. Edelhoch H. & Osborne J.C, (1976), adv. Prot. Chem.., 30, 252.

203. Lowey O.H., reserbrough N.J., & farr A.L, (1951), J.biol. chem., 193, 265.

204. Tanford C., & Roberts G.L., (1952), J.am. chem.. soc., 74, 2509.

205. Laskowiski M.Jr., & scheraga H.A., (1954), J.am, chem.. soc., 76, 6305.

206. Loeb G.I., & scheraga H.A., (1956), J. phys. Chem.., 60, 1633.

207. Galzer A.N., Mackenzie H.A., & wake R.G., (1957), nature (London), 180, 1286.

208. Williams E.J., & foster J.F, (1959), J. am. Chem.. soc., 81, 865.

209. Tyamer Z., & shugar D., (1959), acta. Biochim. Polon., 6, 235.

210. Sam Y., & bovey f.a, (1960), J.biol. chem.., 235 (10), 2818.

211. Wettaufer D.B., edsall J.T., & holling worth B.R, (1958), J.biol. chem.., 233, 1421.

212. Donovan J.W., laskowski M., & scheraga H.A., (1958), biochem.biophys. acta, 29, 455.

213. Yang J.T, & foster J.e, (1954). J.am. chem.. soc., 76, 1588.

214. Tanford E., buzzell J.G., rands D.G., & swanson S.A., (1955) J.am. chem..soc., 77. 6421.

215. Tanford C., & buzzell J.G., (1956), J. phys. Chem.. , 60, 225.

216. Theodore T.H., (1965), J.viol.chem., 240 (2), 628.

217. Saga H.J., & signer S.J., (1962), biochem, L, 305

218. Tanford C. (1962), J. am. Che,. Soc. , 84, 4240.

219. Tanford C., buckley C.E. lively E.P, (1962), J. boil. Chem.., 237, 1168.

220. Bayliss N.S., & mc rae E.G, (1954, J.phys. chem.., 58, 1002.

221. Kay C.M, & edsall J.T, (1956), arch.biochm.biophys., 65, 354.

222. Laskoeski M., widom J.M., mc fadden M.l, & scheraga H.A., (1956), biochm.biophys.acta, 19, 581.

223. Ito M., inuzuka k., & imanishi S., (1960), J.am.chem.soc., 82, 1317.

224. Leach S,J., & scheraga H.A., (1960), J.biol.chem., 235, 2827.

225. Fodter HF., in Putnam W.P (editor), (1960), the plasma proteins, academic press. Inc., new york, chap 6.

226. Nagakura S., & baba H., (1952), J.am.chem.soc., 74, 5693.

227. Pimentel G.C., (1957), J.am.chem.soc., 79, 3323.

228. Nrealey G.J., & kaska M., (1955), J.am.chm.soc., 77, 462.

229. Lars-olov A., (in birgen B. & lars A.H. editors), (1979), plasma proteins, john wiley & sons, pp.43.

230. Agha N.H., Al-illi A.M., & daher N.D., (1985), nukl.mediz., 24 (2), 96.

231. Milo G., (1984), biopharmaceutics and clinical pharmacoknetics. 3rd edition, lea & febiger, chapter 1 and 14.

232. Blok D., feitsma R.I.J., wasser N.j, nieuwenhuizen w. and pauwels. E.K., (1989), nucl,med.biol., 16 (1), 11.

233. Nazar H.A., abdul-miniam A., (1985), report no.6340-pol.85, I.A.E.C.

234. Rae venter B., & dao T.L., (1982), biochem. Biophys.res.commun, 107 (2), 624.

235. Kroesbergen J., gelsema W.J., & delgny C.L., (1986), J. nucl,med.biol., 12, 419.

236. Ortega A., & mas oliva J., (1986), biochem.biophys.res.commun., 139 (3), 868.

237. Olsen S.F., slaninova J., & treiman M., (183), acta.physiol.scand., 118, 355.

238. Sobue K., muramoto Y., fufita M., (1981). Biochem.biophys.res.commun., 100 (3), 1063.

239. Anderson J.R., (1980). Muirs textbook of pathology, eleventh edition Edward arnld.chap.13.

240. Haro L.S, & talamantes F.G., (1985), molec.and cellular endoc, 43, 199.

241. Pires E.M., & parry S.V., (1977), biocem, J., 197, 89.

242. Melander W., & hovarth C., (1977), arch.biochem., biophys, 183, 200.

243. Evans J.S., & Levine B.A., (1980), J. lnorg.bioche,., 12, 227.

244. Cox J.A., malnoe A., & stein E.A., (1981), J.biol.chem., 256 (7). 3218.

245. Kong A.G., Christy B., & Hupf H.B., (1973), J.nucl.med., 14, 695.

246. Backhter M., Al-deen, (1992), phd.thesis, college of science, university of Baghdad.

247. Price P.A., otsuka A.S., poser J.W., kristaponis J., & raman n., (1976), proc.natl.acad.sci.usa., 73, 1447.

248. Hauschka P.V., lian J.B., & gallop P.M., (1975), proc.natl.acad.sci.usa., 72, 3925.

249. Linda A., bhown M., & butler W.T, (1980), J. of boil.chem., 255, 5931.

250. Price P.A., & nishimoto S.k., (1980), proc.natl.acad.sci.usa., 77. 2214, 251

251. Price P.A., & baukol S.A, (1980), J.biol.chem., 255, 11660.

252. Paul P., in William A.P., (authers), (1983), bone & mineral research, annual-1, excerpta medica.

253. Betts F., Blumenthal N.C., posner A.S., becker G.l., & lehninger A.l., (1975), proc.natl.acad.sci.usa., 72, 2088.

254. Price P.A., & nishimoto S.k., (1980), proc.matl.acad.sci.usa., 77, 2234.

255. Poser J.W., esch f.S., ling N.C., & price P.A., (1980), J.biol.chem., 255, 8685.

256. Watkins D., & white B.A., (1985), J.biol.chem., 260, 5161.

257. Poser J.W., & price P.A., (1979), J.biol.chem., 254, 431.

258. Price P.A., parthemore J.G, & deftos L.J., (1980), J. clin invest., 66, 878.

259. Terance G., (1972), the tools of biochem., pp.53.

260. Raddi A.H., & huggins C.B., (1972), proc.natl.aad.sci.usa., 69, 1601.

261. Merk E., clinical laboratory, (1974).

262. Chamberlain J., jargarineen, & ofner P, (1966), biochem.

263. Prince P. A., lothringer J.W., & nishimoto S.k. (1980), J. biochem., 255, 2938.

264. Price P.A., joseph W.L, Sharon A.B., & eadii A.H., (1981), J. biochem., 256 (8), 3781.

265. Pinckerton T.C., ferguson D.l., deutsh E., heineman W.R., & lobson k., (1982), int J.appl.radiat.isot., 33, 907.

267. Garnett E.S., boen B.M., coates G., nahmias C., (1975), invest.radiol., 10, 564.

268. Pietzach H.J., spies h., Hoffmann S., & scheller (1990) int.J.appl.radiat.isot., 41 (2), 185.

269. Hugigen Y.M., gelma W.J., & lignyde C.L., (1987), int. J.appl.radiat.isot, 38, 615.

270. Zodda J.P., tanab S., heinemam W.R., & deutsch F., (1986), int.J.appl.radiat.isot., 37, 345.

271. Leev, W., caldarone A.G.,flak R.H., rubinow A., amd cohen A.S. (1983), radiol., 148, 239.

272. Blumenthal N.C.,& posner A.S., (1987), collodids surfaces, 26, 123.

273. Sehumichen c., rempfle h., wagner M., & Hoffmann G., (1979), eur.J.necl.med., 4, 423.

274. Huigen, Y.M., krips H.j, hulleman S., gelsema w.J., & lagmd. C.L.. (1989) int., J.appl.radiat.isot, MS527.

275. Charkes n.d., (1979), J.nucl.med., 20, 794.

276. Schumichen C., (1984), nukl.mediz., 2, 73.

277. Wilson G.M., & pinkerton T.C., (1985), anal.chem., 57, 246.

278. Schumichen C., kock k., & Kraus A., (1980), J.nucl.med., 21, 1080.

279. Pinkerton T.C., change k.T., show S.M., & witson G.M. (1986), J.nucl.med.biot, 13, 49.

280. Hyghes S., davies R., khan R., & Kelly P., (1978), J.nucl.med., 19, 332.

281. Talmage R.V., matthewas J.i, martin J.ii, kennedy J.w., davits W., royeroft jr,j,ii, (1975), extripta medica, 284.amsterdam.

282. Vanden brand J.A., das H.A., dekker B.G, & lignyde decol, (1982), int.J.appl.radiat.isot., 33, 917.

283. John F.B., (1964), J.am.chem.soc, 86, 4291.

284. Hubbard M.J. & klee C.B., (1987), J.biol.chem., 262, 15062.

285. Agre P., gardner k., & Bennett b., (1983), J.biol.chem., 258 (10), 6258.

286. Gregory A.W., & perry B.M., (1981), life science, 29, 313.

287. Segal H.I, (1976), biochemical calculation, 2nd edd, john willy & sons inc.

288. Kosk-kosicka D., bzdga T., & warzynow A., (1989), J.biol.chem., 264 (33), 19495.

289. Mills J.S., walsh M.P., nemcek k, (1988), nature (London), 330 (6144) 176.

290. Malncik D.A., & Anderson S.R., (1986), biochem, 25, 709.

291. Emil L.S., (1983), principles of biochemistry general aspects, 7th ed mc graw-hill book comp., pp.296.

292. Kauzmann W., (1959), advance port.chem., 14, 1-63.

293. Ross P.D., and Subramanian S., (1981), biochem , 20, 3096.

294. Blumenthal D.K., & stull J.T., (1982), biochem, 21, 2386.

295. Laporte D.C., wireman B.M., & storm D.R., (1980), biochem, 19, 3814.

296. Edelhoch H., & Osborne J.C., (1976), Adv, prot.chem., 0, 183.

297. Weiss B., & Levin R.M., (1978), adv.cyclic nucleotide res, 9, 285.